THE

FLIGHT NURSE

BIBLE

A FIELD GUIDE TO AWESOMENESS

ROBERT P. HARRIS RN BSN
CFRN CTRN TCRN CEN CPEN C-NPT CCRN

LEGAL DISCLAIMER

The content provided in this book is not meant to be a substitute for Professional Advice and is not to be used for ANY Medical Diagnosis and/or Medical Treatment. Medicine is an ever-changing discipline and the Author is not responsible for any negative consequential actions because of omissions and/or errors obtained from the use of the provided content.

You MUST consult, utilize, and follow your CURRENT Policy, Procedure, and Protocol Manuals/Standing Orders. This goes in tandem with additional Radio/Phone Medical Consults or Physician/Medical Director Mandates. This includes relevant Equipment Manufacturer Recommendations. This book and it's contents are not intended as a substitute for any of the aforementioned items.

Additionally, the Author makes no claims whatsoever, expressed or implied, about the superiority of this completed work to the aforementioned items.

To my father Kirk Harris - Legendary Flight Paramedic and Educator Extraordinaire.

To Jennifer Saunders for the Constant- Fun- Sexy Companionship, Flight Nursing Expertise, and Love.

To Christopher Hitchens for teaching us HOW TO THINK.

To Meghan McCool for being a cherished CCT mentor and providing me with a fantasy lifestyle and work environment.

To my brother Samuel Harris for making me want to be someone worth looking up to.

To Lucky, our amazing 24 year old immortal kitten. She was my cuddly study companion for every Cert I have.

To all the Heroes who have given their lives in service of another.

Hello There! Welcome to my Bible!

My name is Robert P. Harris RN BSN CFRN CTRN TCRN CEN CPEN C-NPT CCRN. You can call me Rob, or Nurse Rob if we are being formal. Pleased to meet you! I'm glad you are here. Congratulations on having acquired this Bible! This is the book I wish someone had shown me earlier in my Career! I think you will find this book helpful and accurate. Please have a seat in the front row and we will begin. **Welcome to The Show!**

Just to get my pedigree out of the way: I started my Medical Career as an EMS Explorer at the age of 16. This was a very fun and surreal time in my life. I experienced a sequential series of crazy anecdotal events which inspired and motivated me to achieve success as a Healthcare Provider. Following the devastating 9/11 attacks of 2001, I joined the U.S. Navy to become a Corpsman (Medic). I served in The Iraq War as a "Green Side" Platoon Corpsman with the 1st Marine Division, but that's a long story for another day. A few years later, when I was preparing to leave the Navy, I discovered they allowed Corpsmen to challenge for the LVN (Licensed Vocational Nurse) License. I eagerly took advantage of this opportunity and began working as an LVN in a local San Diego Emergency Department. While working full-time, I went to school for my ADN (Associate Degree in Nursing). After earning my ADN and RN, I worked Registry at various ER's and ICU's, and ran CCT (Critical Care Transport) Ambulance calls. I studied and earned many of my Board Certifications and Course Completions during this time while completing my BSN (Bachelor of Science in Nursing). At my 3-year RN anniversary mark, my resume and experience level were finally ready. I was fortunate and immediately got hired for Flight! I started performing Rotor-Wing (RW)(Helicopter) and Fixed-Wing (FW)(Plane/Jet) Transports. I've been working in Transport Nursing for many years now and have completed thousands of Multidisciplinary Flights/Transports thus far.

 Now before you start rolling your eyes- Please Listen: I'm not trying to compare resumes with anybody! I am simply explaining how I have an experienced Multidisciplinary "Transport-Intensive" background. As a result, most of my thinking, planning, and strategizing is "Transport" centered. Please keep this in mind when evaluating the thoughts, actions, and positions discussed in this Bible.

A few additional disclaimers to get out of the way now:

*- Unless specified otherwise, all roles and titles (Physician,

Nurse, Paramedic, EMT, Firefighter, FLIGHT KNIGHT, Partner, etc.) are gender neutral.

*- I'm going to intentionally not mention the names of specific Dates, Locations, Companies, Hospitals, Agencies, or Individuals. I will alter them as needed for the sake of cogent storytelling.

*- I will use drug names by class/subtype and equipment by function instead of specific brand names. I find this to be a prudent step ensuring the globality of this completed work. You can fill in the blanks based off your own local Protocols and supply. My ideas are intended to be "Tactical and Practical". I might say some "Down & Dirty" things, please meet me halfway and look at the underlying points. My favorite phrase in all of Medicine is "SITUATION DICTATES" (Followed immediately by "DO NO HARM" of course!).

*** - An exception to the above rule will be a brief mention about the value and utility of Ketamine in the modern FlightWorld. Since this drug has been misunderstood and under-utilized for decades, I think it's important to discuss it briefly. I do not have a Crystal Ball telling me what the future will hold for Ketamine Protocols, but this drug presently offers immediate benefits in our Field and I will briefly mention those.

*- A Note to Paramedics, Physicians, and Respiratory Therapists:

While I have the utmost respect for all your integral roles, I am not presently a Paramedic, Physician, or Respiratory Therapist. So out of respect and deference to your skillsets, and for ease of readability and purposes of branding- I will be catering my advice specifically to the "Flight Nurse" role. Please read this book anyway and take away what you want. Most of the material is non-role-specific. Regardless of your Medical background, there will be many take-home thoughts and points worthy of your time. Thank You All!

*- A couple last thoughts before we begin:

Objectively, prayer obviously does not work, or none of us would have jobs!

Planning and Technique Save Lives!

Prayer does not. So, you better TRAIN HARD!

AND

Everybody just Relax. Stay Calm. **TAKE A DEEP BREATH!** Try to responsibly have fun out there. We are all on the same team here. It is us against death! If you are not enjoying life, then you are already dead- Death just hasn't swung by and picked you up yet!

And please learn to smile, you look so much better this way!

 Thank you! Enjoy! And whatever you do -

DO NOT WALK INTO A TAIL ROTOR!

SPECIAL FOREWORD FOR ASPIRING RNs

I want to become an RN, and I think someday I would like to be a Flight Nurse. How do I make this happen?

First things first, become a Nurse! Most Flight Jobs will not consider you for candidacy until you have at least 3 to 5 years Emergency/Critical Care Nursing experience. This means if you want to Fly, you need to shortcut and optimize your Career path. Do not waste valuable time! ADN is the fastest direct route to starting the stopwatch on your Nursing Career. Do not worry about the pedigree of your school. Once you are elite with lots of Certs behind your name no one will ever give a hoot about where you went to school. Sign up for the fastest factory ADN program you can get into, graduate, and pass your "NCLEX" Nursing Board Exam ASAP! Do not worry about student loans! Take them; Use them; Get thru school quickly; Then pay a chill student loan bill every month and don't sweat it. Student loan bills are best viewed as a "Tax On Success". You want a car? You pay a car payment. You want a phone? You pay a phone payment. You want to earn your Nursing Degree in a short period of time and start your lifelong Career with 6-figure income potential? Then take out student loans and shut up! If you have decided to become an RN, then

EVERY DAY you are not an RN you are losing money! Lots of money! EVERY DAY!

(Yeah, yeah, I know. Nursing isn't about the money. It's about the Honor, Integrity, and Privilege of caring for others and leaving a lasting Legacy and all that great stuff. Let's just get on with it shall we? Thank You!)

By the way, let me Congratulate you on choosing to be an RN! Healthcare is the very definition of a growth industry. People have never lived longer, and there have never been so many people! We need you now more than ever! Someone once told me: "Healthcare Is Like A Casino, The House Always Wins!".

Once you pass your Nursing Board Exam and the Career stopwatch has started- You can begin strategizing your future successes. Over the next 3-5 years you can add additional Degrees to your education and Certs to your resume. The goal is to hit your 3-year mark with the most intense resume possible. This will, at the very least, help ensure you are invited to the Flight Interview! Welcome and Goodluck!

THE 12 FLIGHT NURSE COMMANDMENTS

#1: Be Nice

#2: Be Situationally Aware and Prepared For Anything

#3: You Are Only As Good As Your Last Flight

#4: Do Not Get Tunnel Vision: Stop Severe Bleeding - Needle Decompress BOTH Sides of The Chest - Secure The Airway

#5: Take A Deep Breath - Calm Your Voice Tone and Speed

#6: Be A Master of Machines & Know Your Pharmacy

#7: Capnography Is Unimpeachable

#8: Everything Is Your Fault, Document Well

#9: Know When To Gather Your Equipment & Walk Away Slowly and Quietly

#10: Reassess, Reassess, Reassess

#11: Do Not Walk Into Tail Rotors

#12: Be Nice

TABLE OF CONTENTS

PART I - FLIGHTWORLD

CHAPTER 1 : A PLAN FOR SUCCESS - COURSES & CERTS

*

*- If you are already a Flight Nurse you will probably want to skim this Chapter for the parts specifically relevant to your advanced Career goals!

I am an RN and I want to Fly! Now what?

Find mentors! Seek out brilliant inspiring Nurses whom you wish to emulate and pick their brains. If you see a Flight or CCT Nurse in your facility, go out of your way to introduce yourself. Most Professionals will immediately hand you a business card and enthusiastically encourage you to contact them for more information and guidance. If they do not have a card, politely ask for their email or contact info. Don't be shy, we don't mind!

You are going to need to take some Advanced Nursing Courses, read some books, and start studying for Board Certification Exams. Getting dialed in and up to speed will take some time. Good thing you have the rest of your life to do nothing but work, study, train, and learn!

Let's address a technicality now, before we go further. The term "Cert" is an often-misused term, so let's clarify. There are two main classifications of potential "Cert" items. There are sponsored "Board Certification Exams"; Then there are "Course Completion Certificates" given at the end of a class. Board Certifications are globally accepted for post-nominal use and should be the ONLY items actually referred to as "Certs". Course Completions are obviously not mentioned in your official title; Therefore they should be referred to as "Courses". This is a widespread misunderstanding. It drives me crazy!

Ok, now that we are clear on this point, lets discuss some Advanced Nursing Courses either required or at least very recommended for your future job (Strict requirements will obviously vary by employer).

*- I realize by this point most everyone will at least have their BLS card already. I only mention it below for the sake of being thorough.

ADVANCED NURSING COURSES:

- BLS / ACLS / PALS / NRP:

These industry required "Foundational Courses" will be

beneficial every single day. You are required to retake these courses every two years. This is a good thing as it keeps you fresh on new material and changes.

- TNCC:

This more advanced course is usually very enlightening and educational, particularly for first timers. This course is a sort of "Coming of Age Ritual" for Emergency Nurses. Great fun!

- ENPC:

An important class because it gets you thinking in terms of Pediatric Care considerations. This is not intuitive at first. It takes a little bit of time getting used to performing dosage calculation and hands-on skills with Pediatric-sized Pts.

- TPATC:

Ladies and Gentlemen, this is **FLIGHT KNIGHT ACADEMY!** This course is so much fun! You are going to spend a few days surrounded by some of the most experienced Flight Medicine specialists in the World; Picking up tricks and techniques that will make you very slick in the workplace! I cannot recommend this course enough!

BOARD CERTIFICATION EXAMS:

Now we are going to look specifically into "Post-nominally Presentable Board Certifications" to put after your name. These will help you advance your Career and become even more knowledgeable in the high-level intensity Field of Flight and Critical Care Transport Medicine.

- CFRN / CTRN:

The CFRN is the Elite "Feather In The Cap" every Flight Nurse ultimately wants, needs, and dreams about. It means a lot. So does the CTRN. These two exams are very similar in content. However, there is obviously a separate bank of Flight-specific questions for the CFRN. My recommendations for study materials are Laura Gasparis Vonfrolio's 'ICU CCRN Exam Review' (Green Book); Orchid Lopez' 'Back to Basics'; William Wingfield's 'Ace Test Prep'.

- TCRN:

A very Anatomy and Physiology focused exam. Despite this being one of my later Board Certifications, I was humbled at how much I learned and how many light bulbs "Clicked" while studying and preparing for this exam. The recommended study guide from the BCEN will work just fine, as will Kendra Menzies Kent's 'TCRN Exam Review'. Go through them cover-to-cover and be certain you understand every anatomical landmark mentioned, because you will almost definitely see it again on the exam. This fantastic exam properly prepares and educates Nurses for work within Trauma Systems.

- CEN:

A very beneficial Emergency Medicine/ Critical Care exam. It deals with a lot of foundational Anatomy and Physiology. It also uses scenarios you will see day-to-day in any Emergency Department. I recommend this as your FIRST Cert Exam challenge. Mosby's offers two very nice and user-friendly CEN/ Emergency and Transport Prep Books by Renee S. Holleran. Additionally, Vonfrolio's 'CEN Exam Review' (Purple Book) is essential. The abundance of other online/app CEN Exam study materials is overwhelming. My specific book recommendations are a good place to start. Once again- Go cover-to-cover annotating and underlining new and exciting concepts. Make sure you honestly know what every word means! Especially long difficult-sounding words, because you will see them again!

- CPEN:

A fantastic exam to broaden one's daily mindset to the Pediatric Care realm. Subtle assessment skills and Pathophysiological regularities/irregularities will be covered in depth. The ENA sponsored 'CPEN Review Manual' is a wonderful study guide, especially when combined with Scott Deboer's materials. This is a great exam to take following successful completion of the CEN Exam. **One needs to be comfortable with ALL age groups.**

- C-NPT:

A fun and challenging exam. Unlike all the others mentioned, this Cert is available to a variety of Professional Roles (RN, PM, MD, RT). This is not a well-known exam and very few people have this Cert- Which makes having it kind of special and fun! Study materials for this exam are scarce and I suggest going online and seeing what you can find. I realize that wasn't much help, but I struggled finding an abundance of study material and essentially studied blind by "Exam Outline Topics". This was good enough for me to pass. Like I said, go online and you will find some materials out there somewhere.

- CCRN:

Oh goodness! Alright people, this is where things get a little crazy! This exam is very challenging and high level. The same resources I recommend for the CFRN and CTRN will be very beneficial for CCRN. This exam is a brutal assault on your "Knowledge Comfort Zone". You are going to find out a lot about yourself taking this one. Read about my "Methods" in the next Chapter and Good Luck!

*- PARAMEDICS:

There are several specific study guides marketed for the FP-C, CC-P, and TP-C, and I recommend you purchase and utilize all of them. However, all the exam reference materials mentioned above and in the back pages should be on your study shelf! If you know this material, you will be setup brilliantly for exam success!

CHAPTER 2 : CERT EXAM STRATEGY - "NURSE ROB'S METHODS"

Board Certification Exam Testing Strategies:

There are a few key things to remember while preparing for a Certification Exam:

#1- CERTIFICATION EXAMS ARE NOT A TEAM SPORT! If you want to study in a group, this is fine. If you want to have a friend quiz you this is also fine. When the day comes for the exam, you want to ensure you are as calm and undistracted as possible. You are paying a lot of money to sit for this Board Certification, and when you are sitting in front of the computer screen, you are on your own. I recommend you not only go by yourself to the exam, but you don't even tell anyone when your exam is scheduled! People obviously tend to psych themselves out when they know there's pressure to succeed. You can tell people you're studying for the exam, and you'll be taking it soon. This way, if you do not pass, you do not feel embarrassed. If you wish, you may disclose the exam result later, or you can say nothing and leave people with the impression you are taking your time studying.

I suspect a lot of people never take these exams because they are afraid of appearing foolish or silly if they fail.

This is because they already consider themselves to be "Subject Matter Experts". It is detrimental to their egos to imagine failing an exam on subject matter they already have an (Alleged) mastery of. This is Basic Human Psychology. It takes courage to put yourself out there and test your knowledge. Anyone who doesn't respect your attempt to do this, is not a true friend and is probably scared and jealous. A lot of people are gutless cowards who put down Certification Exams for a variety of dumb and lazy justifications. I have a more Honest and Noble approach- "DO YOU THINK YOU ARE IN THE PROFESSIONAL VANGUARD WHERE YOU WORK? DO YOU THINK YOU ARE AN EXPERT IN YOUR FIELD? THEN SHUTUP AND PROVE IT!".

If you do not have the guts to challenge yourself- Then you are just a punk with a Nursing License! Now Focus Up and Go Get Certified!

#2- CARDIAC, RESPIRATORY & HEMODYNAMIC EVERYTHING!!!

If you look up the Exam Content Outlines, available at the respective sponsor sites, you will discover a huge body of exam weight is spent on these few topics. A lot of people misspend valuable study time on "Outlier topics" barely covered on the exam. They fail to study the Critical Core Concepts mentioned above. I am not making this up! Go look at the exam content outline online. It should be obvious what to expect.

#3- STUDY HARD for several weeks leading up to exam week (4-6 minimum is recommended). Make sure you are scheduled off work the day before and the day of the exam. The final week you need to be flying through flashcards with such familiarity you know the answer at a glance. When studying practice exams- Do NOT read the questions first! Read the answer and rationale sections first! Mark, notate, mnemonic, and scribble all over the answer pages so you know what they are looking for, then read the questions. This will help your Brain "Fast-Track" the learning of important facts. This is WAY better than wasting "Brain Power" taking the practice tests, looking at wrong answers, guessing, being wrong, getting frustrated, and having a counterproductive study session!

*- Of course taking practice tests are important, and we are getting to it! Keep Reading!

Once you are two weeks out, it is conditioning time! Now is the time to self-test 50, 75, or 100 questions at a time to build your testing stamina! Then grade your exams and see how you did. Only do this a few times during the final pre-exam week and address knowledge deficits as they appear. If you do too many practice exams, your brain might melt! Ok, now it's the day before exam day! I want you to go for a walk, go to the beach, get a massage, or go to your favorite daytime hangout restaurant and RELAX. Play a game on your phone, or binge watch your favorite show, only taking brief glances at assorted note cards and mnemonic triggers throughout the day. Have a nice protein-filled evening meal and go to bed at a reasonable time. If you have trouble sleeping, investigate OTC sleep aids, as they will help!

*- Do not take any medications for the first time without consulting your Physician. Especially not the night before a very important exam that cost you hundreds of dollars! Seems like common sense..... But Nope…. Nope….Nope (Sighing and shaking head).

DO NOT CRAM! CRAMMING IS BAD! CRAMMING STRESSES OUT YOUR MIND!

The entire point of this section is to systematically prepare you for exam day, so you do not need to cram!

The Night Before-

Before bed make sure your morning is planned out to be stress free. Your significant other knows to give you space; Your dependents are all responsibly cared for; You are confident you know the right place, time, and directions, etc. Have your required papers and forms of identification out and organized. You don't want to be doing a crazy scramble in the morning trying to remember the code to the safe because you have to get your Passport because you forgot your Driver's License expired last week and the new one is still in the mail.

You get the idea. Plan ahead to keep yourself relaxed and focused. There are many other useful tips for exam day, but these are already covered in-depth within the Titles contained in my "Recommended Books" section.

#4- An Alternate Exam Taking Strategy: GRIP IT AND RIP IT! A fantastic approach to taking any Cert Exam is to simply study for a brief week or so and just go take the blasted thing! The second you walk out of the testing center, after (Most likely) not passing, sit down in your car and write down everything you are confused or frustrated about from the exam. Baffling concepts, age group knowledge, pharmacology or vocabulary you didn't know, etc. Most importantly, take a moment to realize you are still alive! The exam didn't kill you! IT'S JUST AN EXAM! Relax, prepare a bit better and go again in a couple short months. You faced the "Cert Exam Dragon" and you lived to fight another day! But now you know how to prepare for the Dragon and what it looks like, which is more than half the battle!

*- Ok, I know some of you are thinking, "Man this is going to be expensive!"- Darn right it's gonna be expensive! You think unimpeachable resumes just appear out of nowhere? No, you got to pay to play! These Cert Exams are worth it. You are going to feel empowered when you pass these exams, and your knowledge level is going to be very heightened..... You are preparing your Brain for the Elite World you will someday encounter at FLIGHT KNIGHT ACADEMY! You will also be

financially compensated and rewarded over time by your employers for the Specialty Board Certifications you hold. They will ultimately pay for themselves many times over. Do not worry about the money! You are making an investment into your Career and Legacy!

I do realize my "Grip It and Rip It" approach to Cert Exams is financially stressful and challenging. Quit your whining and knuckle up! If you want these Certs, you better be in these testing centers every couple months repeatedly until you have the "Post-nominally Dominant" resume you want! NOBODY SAID THIS WAS GONNA BE EASY! You think these exams are hard? Just wait 'til you are intubating a Child on the side of the road in the middle of the night, four Flights and 30 hrs into a 24 hr shift. These Certs are just the beginning. Trust me, its gonna get way crazier! If this didn't just give you a "Thrill-Chill" up your spine, then put this book down and go become a bank teller or something more suited to your lame sense of adventure!

CHAPTER 3 : GOING FOR IT!

Ok, I've been an RN for at least 3-5 years and my resume absolutely rocks! Now what?

Now for the fun part! Job Interviews! Yay! There are several Flight Nurse Career websites out there, some 3rd party recruiters, and some direct company hire. It is time to start applying. Apply hard and fast for every job you can find. Call all your connections and pull all social strings to get your big break. It might take one, two, or ten job application processes to result in your first job. This is normal, don't stress it. Also, do not take it personal. You will most likely never know why you did not get any particular job. This is frustrating but try to intensely self-evaluate your actions and answers during these interviews, pick at things you can improve on, then move on. Do not beat yourself up. There could be dozens of potential reasons why you didn't get picked for a job. Most likely it wasn't personal. Unless you blew it and you know exactly what went wrong. In which case, fix it and try again!

It is important to prepare strategically for job interviews. Be prepared to be dynamic and caught off guard. There are many interview prep websites out there and numerous articles referencing common Flight Interview questions and Scenarios. Please make sure you are familiar with all of them, and practice answering them out loud to your friends, on camera, etc. You will need to be able to perform complex dosage calculations in front of a group of people in real time as they call out numbers. If you have practiced this, it's a piece of cake! If you haven't, then it's a nightmare, and SHAME ON YOU! Depending on how "In over your head you are", there might be required skill demonstrations beyond anything you might have done thus far (RSI (Rapid Sequence Intubation), Surgical Crich, Chest Tubes, etc.). Be honest and if you have never done something, say so! Because they will know from a mile away if you are lying. There are many subtle and tell-tale techniques that will give your inexperience away if you fake it. Just be honest and do not claim to know more than you actually do. Positivity and teachability are most likely what they are looking for anyway. Nobody expects someone who has never flown before to rock a very complex and advanced algorithm under pressure. They know you are Human. They already know you are not perfect. They want to see how you act when you are stumped, frustrated and embarrassed. Even if you are doing everything right and totally owning it, they will keep going until you are stumped and out of good options, because this is the entire point! How do you handle adversity? How does your mind work when all is lost? These hands-on Scenarios and Procedures are far more about seeing your character and composure than actual technical knowledge. If hired, they will see to it you are properly educated on all thing's "Procedure and Protocol". All they really want initially is to see if you are worth their time and money.

Also, just a tip from painful personal experience- Nobody cares how smart you are if you are a cocky jerk! I have seen many jobs awarded to far less qualified individuals because I couldn't find the appropriate mixture of confidence, class, intensity, humility, and arrogance.

*- In fact, I still struggle with this every day, and probably will my entire life. You will too, don't worry! If any of you ever come up with the perfect solution to this "Humility VS Arrogance Equation"- Please let me know first!!!

Ok, enough silliness, lets recap. You have a great resume, you are smart, and you are hungry for a Flight Job. Keep applying. Keep working. Keep networking. If you stay motivated and focused, you will eventually land your first Flight gig. Then the real fun begins!

CHAPTER 4 : YAY! I GOT HIRED! NOW WHAT?

- BOOTCAMP:

Congratulations! You are finally off to FlightWorld bootcamp! Depending upon your company or agency, this is going to be a very different experience for each of you wherever you go. However, there are some general suggestions and tips for success we will discuss.

Bootcamp will most likely be a week, perhaps two. You will spend the first few days getting acquainted with the company dynamics, aviation safety, an entire syllabus of Helicopter-specific topics. This is essentially "Getting you logged in and NOT walking into Tail Rotors", as one of my early mentors so bluntly put it. Then it will be on to Medical and Procedural lectures about anything and everything! You are going to get intense, high-level training throughout the entire bootcamp course, and you better be taking notes and studying your tail off! Because there will be a comprehensive exam at the end of bootcamp- Upon which your job offer depends. That's right, finishing bootcamp doesn't mean you are in, bootcamp is just the start. So listen, study, and be ready to rock the final exam.

Ok, now you passed bootcamp and are checking in for your orientation either at your assigned Base, or you are floating to multiple Bases for orientation. Orientation is by no means universal. Some places have accelerated orientations for individuals with previous Flight experience; Where your orientation is a series of educational checkoffs, additional training modules, and a mandatory amount of Pt contacts and Transports. Other places have mandated orientation periods of 3-6 months, where your employment is conditional until the very end. I don't know what process you will be set into but stay positive and learn from everyone you can. Because very soon, you will be in the REAL WORLD without a preceptor. Your Partner and Pt are going to need you to be a stellar Teammate. Do not let them down!

*- Your Flight lifestyle is going to differ greatly depending upon whether you are hired at a CBS (Community Based Service) or HBS (Hospital Based Service). A CBS gig is typically more Scene-Call intensive and a little wilder and more fun. An HBS is usually still capable of performing scene calls, but mostly does Hospital contract IFT's (Inter-Facility Transports)(Funny Side Note: Really chaotic IFT's are jokingly referred to as "Well-Lit Scene Calls"). HBS jobs are usually chock-full of Hospital

politics and customer service/regulatory agency hoops to jump through, in addition to your CAMTS requirements and other rules/Protocols. Simply put, try to get a CBS gig! Life will be way more fun, but almost any Flight Job is better than no Flight Job! Take what you can get!

*- Another important factor in your job will be the type of shift. 12hr? 24hr? 48hr? Week on/week off? These are all possibilities. If you are doing 12hr shifts, then you are most likely living close to your Operating Base. If you are commuting far distances, longer shifts are not necessarily a bad thing. This means less travel time to meet shift requirements, and more available days to work another job or have a Real Life (If you are THAT kind of person).

CHAPTER 5 : WELCOME TO FLIGHTWORLD

- SETTLING IN AT BASE:

DON'T! Yeah, that's right! Do not get settled in at your Base. **You are ONE big mistake away from being terminated, litigated, killed in an accident, or some combination of the three!** You should be terrified at the Base! You should spend every waking second going over Protocols, doing practice dosage calc, doing gear scavenger hunts, and developing a "Mastery of Machines" (Monitor, Vent, IV pumps, IABP setup, Electronic Charting System, Toaster oven, etc.). Now, if at some point during this craziness you find time to hydrate, nutritionize, and rest- Then consider yourself lucky! Good luck trying to sleep on orientation, realizing any second the call is going to drop, and with no notice or advanced prep you are entering a crazy situation requiring you to flawlessly perform the craziest, most advanced field techniques and complex algorithms possible! So yeah, sleep well friend, sleep well!

I cannot even tell you how many times I would awake, startled in my bed, with an OCD need to look up a Protocol to give me confidence and mental peace so I could drift off back to a light, restless sleep.

Over time, and with a rapid accumulation of insane experiences and training, you will be able to sleep soundly while On-Shift. I promise! It may take a while, years even, but you will eventually become confident in your own abilities. Then you can sleep well and truly rest, but only then.

- BASE LIVING:

There are many different Base configurations you will encounter during your Career: Single/doublewide trailers, Converted homes, Office spaces, Cabins, Furnished hangars, Hotels, Igloos, Bouncy castles, etc.

Base Living means having to play well with others! If you were never on a traveling team in high school or college, and never served in the Military, then you might be in for a rude awakening! Imagine the most annoying thing about the most annoying person you know. Times it by 100, then move in with them. This will give you an idea about what lies in store.
Just a few things off the top of my head:
- Wall-rocking snoring
- Kitchen table finger and toenail clipping
- Potato chip bag crinkling and open mouth chewing

- Flatulation rivaling Pachyderm capabilities
- Public screaming/cursing fights with significant others on the phone or computer
- Dirty towels and clothes left in the bathroom
- Dirty dishes left in the sink
- Appalling personal hygiene
- People "Borrowing" your food without asking
- Intense oppositional political discourse
- Incessant religious ravings

And Worst Of All- VEGANS!

All jokes aside, you are going to need to stretch your nerves to accommodate living with crazy slobs. If you are not laughing right now, then just wait- You will be soon!

*- One of my greatest pet peeves is the inconsiderate crinkling of food bags in-between crunching and chewing. It's not bad enough I have to listen to your crunching and chewing, but then I must hear your hand repeatedly go into the bag and root around for another handful, crinkling away......crinkle crinkle crinkle.......crunch crunch crunch..... crinkle crinkle crinkle.......crunch crunch crunch........crinkle crinkle

crinkle.....crunch crunch crunch ....

AAAAAAAAAGGGGGGHHHHHHHH!!!! No more! No! Stop it! This is why plates, napkins, or paper towels exist! You can dump the contents of whatever food bag onto it and keep the people around you from wanting to strangle you. Whenever I am either teaching a class (And quite often while I am attending one!), I always bring a stack of napkins to place on a table and I tell everyone "I don't care if you eat in class, but I don't want to hear you eat in class, and if anyone in here thought they were going to eat an apple in a closed tight room full of people trying to learn.......FORGET IT! You can chomp your obnoxiously loud food out in the hallway!". I've never understood that about movie theaters- Let's put a couple hundred people in a room together in close proximity, give them all crunchy popcorn and just see what happens! I always feel like I'm part of a Primatology study at the Zoo whenever I go to the movie theater (Which is never).

Don't even get me started on ice chips, almonds, raw vegetables, table chips at Mexican restaurants or people slurping Pho! What is wrong with you people?!?

- COMMUTING TO BASE:

Most likely, you will be driving or otherwise traveling a pretty good distance for your shifts. If you are one of those blessed people Based within easy driving range of home, then Congratulations! But for the rest of us, commuting it is! Commuting sucks, but since we must rationalize it somehow, let us look at the upside. Commuting has a couple unique benefits. #1- You can mentally prepare for your shift and run thru Protocols. #2- You can listen to audio books! I am a busy individual, and I'm going to be honest- I spend all my time working, playing, studying, or trying to catch up on sleep. I don't often get to read books not exclusively full of Medical content. Over the past several years however, I have been ravenously listening to audiobooks, lectures, podcasts, etc. The amount of material I have been through in this medium would probably have taken the term of my natural life to read. I'm talking about dozens and dozens of titles being checked off my literary "To do list"! I can't recommend this obsession enough. You will be proud of yourself for making best use of your time. Additionally, listening to worthwhile media will benefit your Mind and Intelligence greatly.

- MIXED GENDER LIVING CONSIDERATIONS:

I am going to make this brief. We are all adults. We know what is appropriate and what is not. Don't play games with this or be cute, or you will not last long in FlightWorld. All individuals should be in an appropriate state of attire while in ANY public space at ANY time. Particularly when traversing to and from bedrooms to bathrooms and back. Do not create awkward situations where you work. It is rude, distracting, and inappropriate. If you and a colleague want to have an affair, wait 'til you are off shift and off company property, and go be as consensually inappropriate as you want in a hotel room somewhere! But not at the Base! This means not in the Helicopters or Planes either! I know a few of you are smiling now....... Busted!!! Yeah, that's right, no "Hanky Panky" in the Birds! These Helicopters are not 5 Million-dollar love shacks! They are a Professional Workspace. That being said........... Nevermind. Moving on.

- FLIGHTWORLD COMPUTER CHARTING:

You are not going to believe how insane the charting is going to be. The job is amazing, so it is worth it, but Yikes! How bad is it? Real bad. Posting strips, uploading entire digital monitor recordings, uploading Airway Confirmation videos, the insanely inane cutthroat peer review process, long repetitive multistep click button insanity, and Vital Signs every 5 minutes more often than not……. Oh, and by the way, all of this is just for ONE CHART!

Imagine how fun it will be on a busy shift with multiple calls. You will almost never, unless you get skunked, leave the Base on time after your shift. You will be there with your Partner 'til the late morning hammering out the charts. These Flights are typically billed out for anywhere between $10,000-$50,000! So, you can see why they need the chart to be pristine- They are going to have to defend the charges aggressively.

- BASE FOOD:

What you eat at the Base will largely depend on where your Base is located. If you are out in the desert somewhere stranded in the scorching hot wilderness, you will want to eat lots of salads, veggies, fruit, lean protein, and hydrate like a beluga whale! In extreme heat, heavy meals and excessive comfort food will run you down and make you feel even more miserable. If you are in colder or even normal climates, you might be able to enjoy indulging in heavier courses and perhaps even a reasonable amount of comfort food. I am pretty low maintenance myself, I usually keep an assortment of prepackaged deli lunchmeats and salads in the fridge/cooler. This accompanies my leaning tower of assorted canned soups- Which I open and eat with a spoon out of the can with my bottle of hot sauce. Delicious! What can I say?...... I'm a man of simple tastes I suppose.......ELEGANCE IS A STATE OF MIND!

- BASE HYGIENE:

Trust me, you stink! No, seriously, you stink bad! Nobody wants to be the stinky pig-pen person. Please rinse off at respectable intervals and keep your dirty laundry in tied or sealed plastic bags out of courtesy for the next person who must use your room. BRING YOUR OWN SPRAY DISINFECTANT CAN! There are many wonderful products out there, specifically designed to keep you from being a stinky disgusting mess! Soap is not a scary new potion we are "Tar and Feathering" Witches for inventing! It has been around in various forms and civilizations for quite a while! Please use some! Trust me, if you can't think of who the smelly person is at your Base, then it is you, Congratulations! Now go buy some soap! Seriously, right now!

CHAPTER 6 : ALL THINGS NARCOTICS

- NARC CONTROL/ ACCOUNTABILITY:

This is going to vary State to State, County to County, City to City, Agency by Agency, etc. In most of my personal experience the RN has maintained possession of the narc box. Or the RN and PM both have smaller narc boxes. In a perfect FlightWorld, the call drops, and the crew prepares to lift and the Flight Crew (RN-RN or RN-PM) does a dual person narc lockbox checkout, sometimes with separate keys like an old soviet nuclear submarine movie. Or sometimes with bio-scanners of an ever-assorted variety. Once the narcs are out, then what? They go in secure pockets on someone's person until it is time to remove an already pre-selected and agreed upon specific medication and dosage. The vial should remain in plain view whenever feasible (Unless the situation clearly dictates otherwise- Emergently drawing up a "Benzo" to stop a seizure in turbulence at night while your Partner has their hands full performing other Pt care tasks would be an example of when this accountability Procedure MIGHT be suspended, maybe). Then the drug is drawn up from the vial in plain sight and the amount is verified; The administration is performed per

Protocol; The empty syringe is discarded or whatever per Policy.

- THE "NEW PARTNER NARC TALK":

At the beginning of every shift with a new Partner, RN or PM, I make sure we openly discuss Narcotic Accountability. I have a very well-practiced speech I give:

"Ok, real quick, I'm just going to get this out of the way now. I will not give a med without discussing with you first, and we will agree on the dose. Then I will draw up the med and have you verify the amount before administering. I will do this every time for every med. I also am going to ask you to do the same thing with me and make sure I am involved in every Medication Administration you perform. This way you can trust me, and I can trust you. Because let's face it, you and I don't truly know each other very well yet. Cool?".

*- I then always follow up with an additional bit I took from my Flight Paramedic Father: "Two more things- #1. If we have a problem or disagreement, we will call Medical Direction for guidance or we will discuss it later AWAY from the Pt.

#2. PLEASE DON'T LET ME DO ANYTHING STUPID!

I have rarely met anyone who wasn't receptive and appreciative of this necessary conversational gesture. It is a great way to address a touchy subject without being authoritarian, condescending, or self-righteous. Try the speech out, and make sure you are using a polite and cordial tone. Your Partner will at least recognize, if not appreciate, your thoroughness and "Attention to detail". Also, and most importantly, your Partner will think twice before pulling any "Tricks" on you. It makes a very important statement. I cannot recommend this enough! Try it out next shift!

*- This is not being "Cynical". This specific issue is a known problem in Healthcare. This is ensuring necessary Pt and Crew safety. This is not cynicism, it's Professionalism!

- NARCOTIC POLICY, ABUSE, AND DIVERSION:

It happens everywhere. Be mindful. It could be your best friend. The signs are usually tell-tale, or at least mildly eyebrow raising. Lots of trips to or excessive time spent in bathrooms; Atypical lethargy; Difficult to rouse; Slurred speech/missed words; Motor skill degradation; Always being authoritative and possessive during narc med admin Procedures; Cracking vials without you (That's a biggie!); and ANYTHING ELSE causing an "Honestly suspicious" feeling in your gut.

- BEWARE OF "THE NARC VIAL SWITCHING TRICK":

Ok, this is how the trick is performed. I have been fooled by this trick myself, so I am hyperaware for the tell-tale behavior. Your Partner will be packaging or interacting with the Pt On-Scene, At Bedside, or even Enroute. Then they might suggest, or might wait for you to suggest, analgesia of some variety. Your Partner will then open the narc box and immediate select a particular med and pop the cap off. They might even "Clumsily" drop the vial and scramble for it. All the while talking to the Pt, asking you a question about dosing, or apologizing creatively for their "Accident". They also might apologize for "Mis guessing" the drug they thought "You prefer to use". They will then draw up the med from the vial and administer it seemingly per Protocol. Then they will either pocket the narc box, or possibly return it to you- Making sure to show and tell you the empty vial is in the box! Which it is.

That's it. That's what happens.

Did you catch it? I didn't at first either. My Partner had a used vial of the medication of choice pre-filled with Saline! The trick was where he would make the switch. He would either do it while going into a suit pocket for an alcohol prep or a needle to draw it up or something, or when he "Accidentally" dropped it on the ground.

So, what I was watching was my Partner craftily swap a Saline filled vial for the REAL narc vial, then draw up and administer Saline. You might think- "Wouldn't the lack of effect on the Pt be a red-light-warning suspicion indicator?" Absolutely right! Which the Partner would then brush off as the Pt having a "Strong tolerance", and then would administer an actual "Second" narc dose to suspend suspicion and "Keep them quiet".

When it happened to me, I had suspicions but no actual evidence, and my Partner wasn't acting impaired or "Under the influence". So, we continued the call and the Pt received quality care for the duration with no adverse events. Afterwards, I told him I suspected him of narcotic theft and I demanded an explanation. Surprisingly, my Partner broke down crying and admitted to everything immediately. I was floored! I told him he has to self-report or I was going to be forced to report him. I told him I know Partners need to trust each other, but he had already violated our trust, and the only way to protect myself was to report him. I told him, without apology- "I Do Not Take Chances With My License!". Once we returned to Base he called our Supervisor and gave a full confession and resignation. Incident reports were filled out and then my story became an anecdote in a lecture about "Red Flags" in the workplace. Consequentially, I have never fully trusted any Partner ever since. I may, if you are worthy, trust you with my Life, but never with my Wife, and certainly NEVER WITH MY NARC BOX!!!

CHAPTER 7 : IT'S ABOUT LEGACY

- DEFENDING YOUR SPOT:

Every single shift is a ready opportunity to destroy your Legacy and ruin your Career!

If you do not show proper respect for safety, training, and proper technique, you are a ticking timebomb. We all just hope you don't take anyone else with you when you explode.
Even after you are off orientation, or after your 1st, 5th, 10th, or 20th year Flight anniversary- You are just as susceptible to making a critical screwup and getting yourself or others killed. Quite possibly even more susceptible! You are never safe from the consequences of your actions as a Healthcare Provider. Your Life's Legacy will only be cemented once you're dead. Until then you must fight every day for Honor and Respect. If you live and work every day attempting to be the best Healthcare Provider possible, your Legacy will take care of itself.

There are many people out there who are very caring and kind Healthcare Providers that aren't exactly going to be winning any "Genius Awards" any time soon.... You all know who I am talking about - You are already thinking of at least 3 Coworkers right now before the end of this sentence. Just because you are a Genius doesn't mean you are empathetic to your Pts and help them feel as good as possible throughout their crisis. I know Colleagues who can't even spell the word "Genius", but they care and connect with people on a personal level and their Pts love them.

The Pt is likely only going to remember a few tidbits in memories from their Traumatic Experience. Details will be blurry, actions distorted, but the emotions they had while in your care will always stick with them. Ask yourself honestly- "How did you make your last Pt feel?"; "Are you proud of yourself?"; "Are you ashamed?". Whatever you are feeling right now, dwell on what you can do to be better. Yes, We Can Always Be Better At Something. **Always.**

PART II - HELICOPTER HOW TOs & FLIGHT KNIGHT PROTOCOL

CHAPTER 8 : HOW NOT TO GET KILLED

*- 3 TO GO, 1 TO SAY NO! -

This might be the most important thing in this book! There will come a time where you will have to turn down a Flight because of safety reasons. There will be times where life is on the line and you will have to say no! This is going to emotionally kill you, but disobeying Safety Regulations will physically kill you. THE MOST IMPORTANT PERSON TO KEEP ALIVE IS YOURSELF! The Flight Crew's safety is always priority. I want to be a Hero! I hope a "Heroes' Death" will find me someday! This job is dangerous, I accept that! I am not afraid of death! I dream of glory! BUT if it comes down to my safety and the safety of my Crew against your life- I WILL SEND FLOWERS! We are Professional Lifesavers! What good are we to anybody dead? Please be smart and safe out there! Listen to the "Inner Voice" telling you "This Is A Terrible Idea". There will come a time where you will be asked to break rules, and you will be threatened with disciplinary action or worse. When this happens, and trust me it will, I hope you have the courage to say no. Then I want you to pack up your stuff, get in your car, and go home to your family and appreciate being alive. I'm not afraid of dying, I'm really not, why would I be? I just don't want to die stupidly because a gung-ho psycho Pilot or jerk Supervisor made me go on a Flight with weather moving in and end up slamming into a hillside at 100 knots! If you think I'm being dramatic then you don't know this business very well and you have no idea what you are talking about. The danger is real people! Try not to get killed. LIVE TO SAVE ANOTHER DAY!

CHAPTER 9: SHUTTING DOWN VS HOT LOADING

During your Pilot briefing- Have a pre-discussed plan with your Pilot and Fellow Crewmember about strategies involving communication On-Scene regarding shutting down the Bird (Cold Loading) or keeping it running for an expeditious departure (Hot Loading). Usually, during the day, and with good ground radio communication- Enough Pt information has been exchanged prior to setting down On-Scene for the Pilot and Flight Crewmembers to already have a plan.

*- Do not forget- Operational Safety is our #1 Priority. Do not hog the radio while circling over the Scene attempting to get more Pt info. Assist your Pilot by spotting obstacles and ensuring a safe LZ (Landing Zone). If you get Pt info, then great! But don't stress it. Stay Calm. Land Safely. Then you can go get all the Pt info you want.

At night, or anytime we would walk away and "Assess the situation", I would communicate back to the Pilot or the Tail Rotor Guard with simple hand/arm signals.

Daytime: Throat slice hand = Shut it down; Hand spinning circle motion = Keep it running.

Nighttime: Red Lensed Flashlight waving Side to Side = Shut it down; Red Lensed Flashlight waving in a Circle = Keep it running.

*- The Red Lensed Flashlight is to avoid further damaging your Pilot's night vision with unnecessary white light (Duh!).

Situation Dictates what we ultimately decide to do, but the very general guideline is >10 - 15 minutes = Shutdown.

*- If landing directly on a blocked freeway, the Pilot will most likely want to keep it running, because there is always a chance the Bird will "Hot Start" (Potential Engine Malfunction Alarm during startup sequence) and then we are out of service, not going anywhere, and we are blocking a freeway. Perfect!

No kidding, I have firsthand stories of Pilots being stuck on closed freeways and taping a blanket, window sunscreen, or ANYTHING over the Helicopter logo to decrease company embarrassment when pictures end up on the Evening News and social media. Smart. Very smart.

CHAPTER 10 : BATTERY POWER & OXYGEN

If you run out of either of these two items, your day just took a dramatic turn. Obstacles can be overcome and solutions improvised, but if you run out of O2 in the middle of nowhere and your Pt was dependent upon it.... guess what..... that's right!....ACLS and Incident Reports, because you are stupid! Oh wait, I said ACLS- But your Partner didn't swap out the batteries after the last call and the charger hasn't been working right because you are waiting for a part to arrive at the Base. Now you are trying to analyze ACLS rhythms and code your hypoxic Pt, but you don't have a monitor because the batteries are dead! And of course, the Pilot is unable to reset the inverters to get you more power, but it doesn't matter because you don't have the cable anyway, and even this doesn't matter because without any O2 your vented Pulmonary Pt has ZERO chance of resusc.......... Aaaaaaaaaaaaaahhhhhhggggg!!!

Now, could any of this have been avoided?

Ummmm......Freakin Duh!!!

Do not go on ANY Flight unless you are very certain you have MORE THAN ADEQUATE amounts of BATTERY POWER and O2. Fortunately, I have not been in the drama of the situation above, but very early in my Career a coworker was.

They are no longer actively working in the industry, and this is probably best. Seeing firsthand the fallout from this "Mega-Disaster" scared me straight! I proudly declare myself neurotically OCD about BATTERY POWER and O2! I hope you also become afflicted by this passionate desire to not become a cautionary tale.

It is imperative you know how to troubleshoot electrical issues in your Bird. This should be part of any standard orientation with each new Transport Vehicle you encounter. Have the Pilot walk you through the Inverter Reset Procedures, because many of these electrical systems need to be manipulated in a series of complex steps. Or maybe it's just one switch and you go "Click". I don't know what it will be for you, hence the point of the exercise.

- SETTING DOWN IN THE MIDDLE OF NOWHERE WITH A PT ONBOARD:

Ok, something went wrong, and now you are in "Booneyville", out in a field at 0300 with no idea 'what's what' and 'where's where'. Get on the radio/phone with your "Dispatch Hub" and get in touch with the closest EMS Provider. You will need them to show up with a rig, because you will most likely need more Battery Power or O2 at some point. Also, request the launch of another Bird to come help "Salvage The Situation" and continue Transport! Begin to strategize an "Extended Pt Treatment Plan" and prepare for the ever-impending Worst Case Scenario (WCS).

- EQUIPMENT CHECKS:

- Daily at least, morning and evening recommended

- Monitor Defib Check

- Thorough Med Bag Inventory

- Enough O2?

- Enough Battery?

- Inverter and Plugs Functioning?

- Charging Cables for ALL gear present and intact?

- Behavioral Restraints easy access? (It's Gonna Happen Quick!)

*- Put Zippers on all equipment bags either in the middle or on the particularly appropriate side for easy "In-Flight" access.

This might sound trivial but trust me- Extra stress and irritation caused by an inability to reach zippers while scrambling for a piece of gear in the middle of the night while the World is ending around you is something to be avoided.

- THE OCD BAG COUNT:

This is a way to ensure you never leave anywhere without ALL your equipment. This is important for a ton of obvious reasons. As silly as it sounds, it is surprisingly easy to forget equipment and leave something behind. Either in a Trauma Bay, on a Hospital rooftop, back at the Base in the middle of the night, etc. If you develop a numbering system or a literal CHECKLIST- Then YOU WILL NEVER FORGET A PIECE OF EQUIPMENT! 1, 2, 3, 4, 5………Dangit! I forgot the O2 Tank in the corner of the Trauma Bay- I gotta go back down and get it before we lift from the rooftop. No big deal. Self-inflicted "Screwup Crisis" avoided! Writeups and Incident Reports avoided! Yay! OCD is a virtue in Healthcare. Take my word for it.

CHAPTER 11 : FIRE BAD

- CRASH RESISTANT FUEL SYSTEMS, JET FUEL, AND BURNING TO DEATH:

Ok, here is the sad tragic reality: If you are fortunate enough to survive a hard set down or crash landing- Your next immediate greatest concern, and worst fear is burning to death. Many organizations have yet to convert their platforms to a CRFS (Crash Resistant Fuel System)(Non-rigid, flexible fuel bags are WAY less likely to burst and leak on impact than a rigid plastic or thin walled aluminum fuel tank). I know there may not be much you can do to change the fuel tank situation at your present workplace- But please **"Beware The Danger"**. Advocate/recommend greater Safety Compliance whenever possible. Governmental regulations will eventually ensure a CRFS is the mandated industry standard, but this will take years, even decades. So please be careful, wear appropriate safety equipment, and be very familiar with the egress strategies in your Bird. Any internet image/video search will provide you with many disturbing/nightmarish examples and case studies on this point. Many members of our Flight Family and their Pts have suffered excruciating fiery deaths unnecessarily. All because some company somewhere wanted to save some money. If this doesn't make you furious, then Read It Again! Because it should!

*- I am sorry to bring down the mood and get all militant about this morbid topic, but it hits me on a personal level and really pisses me off. **Let us take a moment of silence for the Fallen**...............

Ok, now then, let us continue our discussion like Professionals.

- FLAME RETARDANT FLIGHTSUITS:

They work, so wear them properly. Long sleeves required. Unfortunately, in some excruciatingly frustrating physics-based irony, flame retardant Flightsuits are made of very special chemically woven fabric that is stifling hot in summer holding air in and paper thin cold in winter allowing wind right through. It sucks for those of us who operate in harsh climates but it's just part of the game. Note: Be sure to carefully launder your Flightsuits per manufacturer specs or you might damage the integrity of the suit's fire-retardant properties.

A brief internet search will yield numerous images demonstrating the difference in degrees of Burn Trauma With VS Without flame retardant materials. These images are impressive and terrifying.

For coats and undergarments, you want to avoid wearing synthetic fabrics! In the event of a fire, they "Flash Melt" and adhere to your body, encasing the affected regions in a "Plastic Lava Blanket".

- COTTON, COTTON, COTTON!!!

Cotton still burns, but when it lights up, it (Somewhat) protects your skin from the flame and burns to ash instantly, not Plastic Lava.

CHAPTER 12 : OTHER SAFETY EQUIPMENT

- HELMET VISORS:

They need to be down whenever feasible. If you have ever experienced a Bird Strike- Then this is self-evident! You can get very injured kissing a Seagull, Red-Tailed Hawk, Sparrow, Bat, or Raccoon at 100 knots. Protect your face!

- EYE PROTECTION:

I always recommend having your corneas protected when performing any Flight Operation- day or night. Have a nice pair of close-fitting wraparound sunglasses you hang around your neck, so they do not get lost. Personally, I prefer exotic tinted lenses (Especially Red!). They make life more fun! If you are a boring person and no fun at all then just get plain old dark tint (Yawn).

Then get yourself a comfortable pair of wrap-around clear-lens glasses for night time corneal protection, it also serves as additional- Already in place BSI (*- Not a substitute for actual BSI Precautions!). Keep them in your onboard Personal Flight Bag, or Flightsuit pocket in a compact rigid case for scratch protection and rotate your day time sunglasses out for the night time pair when appropriate. Also, there are many cool options out there with tints and built in lights. Fun!

- HEARING PROTECTION FOR CREW:

Huh? What did you say?

It's simple Science- Large amounts of extreme noise level exposure over time results in permanent hearing damage (No really?!?). It is intelligent to wear some sort of low-profile ear insert (In addition to your helmet) to protect your hearing during Flight Operations. As long as your ability to communicate is not impeded. There are also several cool in-helmet "Noise-cancelling" products on the market worth investigating.

- HEARING PROTECTION FOR PTS:

We also need to PROPERLY protect our Pt's hearing. In-ear rubber or foam plugs are useful, or perhaps your platform is furnished with industrial grade ear muffs or radio headsets. Either way, it is a nice consideration and will help keep your Pt calmer and more relaxed. This is particularly important in your comatose/lightly-sedated intubated Pts- Because earplugs help decrease their "Rousability Threshold".

- WATER SAFETY:

The only good thing about a water landing is the decreased likelihood of burning to death. Drowning? Possible, sure, but burning? Probably not. If your organization operates in and around large bodies of water routinely, it is likely you will undergo some sort of Underwater Vehicular Egress Training. This training is intimidating and intense. The intensity will vary by program. Anything from treading water in a pool with your Flightsuit and boots on while manually self-inflating a life vest; To being restrained in a mock vehicle with a half dozen other people and dropped into a pool and forced to systematically egress appropriately. If your training is as intense as the latter, then you are in for some real fun! Do not worry! They have divers standing by with air in ready supply and they are watching all of you very carefully. Does this make the experience any less terrifying? No. Not at all, it is crazy scary, but very necessary and rewarding. Seeing how efficiently you can egress calmly while underwater seems daunting, but the experience is intended to Promote Survival and the ability to Remain Calm under pressure. There will be many unknown variables to any water landing. This means any training performed is probably not going to fully prepare you for a realistic near-drowning crash experience. Some of those variables are: Day or night; Type of airframe (Clamshell vs side entry, etc.); Water temperature; Weather calm or storming; Helicopter "Floatie" buoyancy devices or not; Angle and speed of water entry; etc. So... is it beneficial to undergo water egress training? Sure, of course! Why would you not? But just mentally prepare yourself for the likely reality of a very bad outcome in the event of such an event.

IF YOU ARE NOT WILLING TO DIE DOING THIS JOB, THEN MAYBE YOU SHOULD STAY HOME WHERE IT'S SAFE.

- HELMETS ON-SCENE?:

If your company has a specific Policy- Follow It!

*- This Bible is just a "Field Guide" filled with tips and practical advice. Do not start a war with your company or a particular Pilot or Crewmember over this......... Just "Go With The Flow" (As long as the "Flow" wants to come home alive!).

Personally, I find myself very stifled and inhibited while wearing a helmet On-Scene. I do not understand why one would need too. It doesn't keep you any safer! The only real threat out there should be getting hit by your own Helicopter. Your helmet is not gonna make any difference if you walk into the Main Disc or Tail Rotor. With or without it, you're gonna become "Human Confetti". The purpose of these helmets is to protect our cranium in a Helicopter crash! NOT to protect from "Fall Down Go Boom" (FDGB) On-Scene incidents. Think about it for a second...... What point is there to walking around On-Scene looking like an awkward "Ricky Rescue" bobble-head? Being helmeted On-Scene makes it more difficult to hear report and decreases your peripheral vision and "Situational Awareness". You also risk damaging or soiling it when/if you set it down. VERDICT: Leave your helmet SECURED in the Bird and go On-Scene uninhibited.

- SECURING EQUIPMENT:

Everything not clamped or tied down well is a potential projectile. Anybody ever been in a MVC? In a storm at sea? Severe turbulence on a Commercial Flight? Yeah..... imagine that, but potentially way worse. **Secure your toys or get skewered!**

CHAPTER 13 : WINKING AT DEATH & CONFRONTING MORTALITY

I'm going to make this quick. Every Human Being on Earth is part of a "Higher" primate species named Homosapiens. Homosapiens, just like all other species of Mammal, are "Warm Blooded Flesh-Suits Full Of Meat And Bone". We are susceptible to the Laws of Physics, whether we like it or not. In other words, we are very "Fragile Critters"!

Oh sure, as Individuals we are capable of amazing feats of strength and ability- But a lot of good that's going to do any of us when faced with Highspeed MVC's, Bipolar Polar Bears, BASE Parachute Failures or Mothers-in-Law!

I'm not trying to be defeatist or nihilistic here. Quite the opposite in fact. I'm attempting to "Mentally Approach Death" as Sensically, Calmly, and Rationally as possible.

There are many easy solutions to common death causes:

- Increase vehicular following distance.

- Don't text and drive.

- Stop smoking.

- Lose some weight.

- See your Physician routinely.

- Put on your seatbelt.

- Look BOTH ways before crossing the street!

And these are just a few quick examples off the top of my head!

The failure of our fellow Homosapiens to follow the guidelines mentioned above will be responsible for TENS OF MILLIONS OF DEATHS within the next year! Yet each one of us will finish reading this paragraph and go on about our day taking one or more of the above survival tips for granted.

So What Does This Mean?

It means we should "Respect" our fragility as Human Beings, but not let this "Respect" cripple our ambition. Experience your life!

Have adventures! Be exciting! Enjoy testing the boundaries of your mental and physical abilities.

It would be a shame to waste this cool "Body-Machine" of ours. Just reflect upon this fact: The Neuro-Chemical Processes and resulting Sympathetic Responses guiding your mental and physical adventures are the cumulative result of MILLIONS of Generations of Biological Evolution on Earth.

(If this irrefutable fact of Science did not just make the hair on your arms stand up- Read It Again! Because its 100% True! **Look it up for yourself!**)

Yeah Nurse Rob, that's great and all- But again, What Does All This Mean?

Do not excessively concern yourself with the fear of death. The day before you were conceived by your parents, were you suffering and miserable because of your lack of existence? No! So why do you think returning to that prior state of non-existence at the end of this life will result in agony and torment? Silly right? Think about it.

Most likely, the only reason you are actually "Afraid" of what

happens when you die is because of some completely unsubstantiated man-made myth or superstition which you grew up believing. Well forget that silly nonsense! You will be better off throwing it away and thinking for yourself!
I PROMISE YOU.

Use your mind.

Live intelligently. Attempt to make more smart decisions than dumb ones. Be kind to each other, and enjoy your precious time on Earth.

PART III : SPECIAL MEDICAL SITUATIONS

CHAPTER 14 : BABY-JITSU

*- Make sure you have an OB Kit in your gear! Scare away the Voodoo! I don't care if you just saw it recently, put "Eyes on" at the start of every shift! Because the one day you don't...... guess what's going to happen!

As a self-respecting modern Healthcare Professional, I understand there is no fate and no intellectual credence given to superstition. BUT!- There are certain things you can do to keep the "Crazy Calls" from going off the rails! That is the ENTIRE point of this Bible!

You really do not want to deliver a Baby In-Flight! There are Helicopter platforms offering limited access to birthing-friendly positioning, but they are few and far between. If you are a bendy individual and can perform "Jiu Jitsu" style maneuvers, then sure, I suppose you can find a position to deliver a Baby. But most likely, vision and clearance are going be obscured dramatically. Not to mention the safety concerns with being unsecured while performing "Baby-Jitsu" during Helicopter Operations. This is not even getting into WCS about Mother or Baby instability or complications. Now you have 2 Pts! And you better be able to provide "Standard of Care" treatment admirably for both! Obviously, this situation is to be avoided at almost any cost! Follow your Protocols and ask specific WCS questions at your company sponsored training sessions. Have Senior Flight Crewmembers and the Medical Directors weigh in on strategies for avoiding inopportune deliveries In-Flight during the Emergent Transport of the Mother. Most companies are NOT going to have active policies in place for Emergency C-Section, so just forget it. Unless it is a crazy-"You happen to know there are Triplets and the Mother is coding, and you have Physician Medical Control on a recorded line talking you through the craziest next 5 minutes of your life"- kind of situation. Outside of that wildly improbable WCS, focus is going to be on Maternal Resuscitation. Perhaps Protocols and Standing Orders will expand in the future, including more aggressive field C-Section techniques. But alas, at this relatively young stage in FlightWorld history- This simply is not reality. So, make every attempt to chemically delay delivery per Protocols and divert to the "Closest Appropriate Facility" (Even if it's by Ground Ambulance!). Otherwise, its "BABY-JITSU" time!

CHAPTER 15 : CPR & ACLS - THE NOBLE DANCE

- NON-TRAUMA CPR:

We need to have a "Thumper" (Mechanical Chest Compression Device) in the Bird! Quality CPR and appropriately safe Helicopter Operations/Crew Resource Management (CRM) are quite often incompatible. It is a challenge to perform quality "Textbook" resuscitation in a sterile Hospital environment with a full team of Professionals, and we are doing it as a 2-person tag team in a flying closet in the dark. Meanwhile, during this chaos, we are "Required" to remain seat-belted for approach and landing, look around for Air Traffic, and assist the Pilot as needed. I have coded in a Helicopter a few times unfortunately (My first was a severely Hypothermic V-Fib Arrest, and a couple other unavoidable Trauma deteriorations ...... a mentor of mine calls these "Character Building Flights"). Of course, we do the best we can, and we get the job done. However, it would be nice having an extra set of CPR-Performing "Robot Hands" making life a thousand times easier! So yeah, we need a "Thumper" in the Bird.

- TRAUMA CPR:

CPR is what we do to prove our devotion to life once someone is dead. It is an obviously necessary and worthwhile practice. At the very least it partially insulates us, and the Pt's loved ones from feelings of helplessness or hopelessness. Knowing "Everything Was Done That Could Be Done" is Psychologically empowering to those involved in Trauma Resuscitation. Because the simple fact is a lot of your Pts cannot be saved. Unfortunately, Trauma Codes in the field don't make it. They just don't. Too much multisystem damage and blood loss. Their only chance is RAPID TRANSPORT to a Trauma Surgeon. Even then, they better still have Vital Signs! The Surgeons cannot make bricks without clay! I am certain future technological innovations will allow for very sophisticated and much more invasive Field Surgical Procedures and Protocols, but we are just not there yet.

There are BILLIONS of People on Earth and not even one of us is getting out alive! If you make caring for the sick and injured your chosen profession, you can naturally expect a good deal of death to happen in your presence. **The old EMS adage goes: "You can't kill a dead guy". Yeah, that's true, but if you suck at your job you are certainly going to help a few out the door.......**

CHAPTER 16 : ALL BLEEDING STOPS EVENTUALLY.........

- MASSIVE HEMORRHAGE- EXTREMITY:

STOP THE BLEEDING! I don't care how you do it! Stop it! Tourniquet practice should be a real thing.

- MASSIVE HEMORRHAGE- NON-EXTREMITY:

JUNCTIONAL and TORSO TOURNIQUET designs are becoming more and more sophisticated and should be stocked and carried. They can also be moderately well improvised with "Proper Prior Planning" and training. There are a lot of different products and devices out there, but the underlying premise is the same- Apply "Crazy-Intense Pressure" to the site of the JUNCTIONAL WOUND and reinforce as well as possible. Then Rapidly Transport!

- MASSIVE HEMORRHAGE- INTERNAL:

Get them to a Trauma Surgeon as expeditiously as responsibly possible. "Supportive Care" per Protocols in the meantime (Txa, Fluids, Blood Products, Pressors, etc.).

*- Be mindful of "Permissive Hypotension" guidelines in Trauma and follow them per Protocols. You just need a "Good Enough" SBP/MAP in these cases.

*- I predict in the future, REBOA (Resuscitative Endovascular Balloon Occlusion Of the Aorta) will be a "Field Skill". It's basically a Femoral Arterial Line with an inflatable balloon to occlude lower Aortic blood flow and prevent exsanguination. Too cool! Someday. Not yet, but someday!

CHAPTER 17 : A SCENE TRIAGE TALE - "SO THIS ONE TIME......"

- MULTI-PT SCENE TRIAGE:

Most of the time when you are responding to multi-vehicle MVC, you will be called in for a specific Pt, and will not be tasked with triage. However, there will be occasions in your Flight Career where you will be the first or nearly the first Medical unit On-Scene. The Procedure is to communicate with your ground contact person (If applicable); Perform a safe landing; Shut down or stay running as per situation; Then check in with the IC (Incident Commander) for further orders and Pt designation. I have been On-Scene on a few occasions where things were not nearly that organized yet, and there had been no triage performed. "So This One Time", My Partner and I begin triaging with the Ground Agency Personnel, expediently hunting for "The Sickest Pt". We knew there were at least a couple of additional Birds on their way, so we were to find "The Sickest Pt" and roll out towards the Trauma Center ASAP! There were a few vehicles, and about a dozen total Pts involved. We began searching the scene and wreckage for Pts. There were quite a few. An SUV with an entire (Mostly unrestrained napping) family had run off the road and rolled-crashing into oncoming traffic. There was an ejected Pt with VERY "Obvious Lividity" which we briefly evaluated then moved on. Ultimately, we found the bulk of the seriously injured in the flipped SUV. There was a teenage girl laying in the back on the ceiling of the SUV, screaming to a Firefighter. My Partner was on the other side of the vehicle talking to another hyperverbal and sobbing occupant. This man ended up being both the father of the family, and the driver who ran off the road and overcorrected, causing the crash. He had self-extricated and was self-splinting an obvious deformity closed LT Humeral Fx. There were a couple other minor injuries, but nothing Critical. THEN WE FOUND GRANDMA! Grandma had fortunately been restrained correctly. She was hanging upside down in the front passenger seat of the inverted SUV wreckage. She was conscious, moaning in pain, and guarding her abdomen with her one good arm. She was covered in abrasions, and had a severely deformed compound RT Humeral Fx which was bleeding profusely. She also had a deformity and severe ecchymosis to her RT Clavicular region and RT infero-lateral Ribcage. She was soaked in blood, and it was pooling on the floor beneath her head. I yelled over to my Partner and said, "I got our Pt! We are taking Grandma! She is clearly on blood thinners and is really banged up!". My Partner came over and instantly nodded his agreement. We began expeditiously extricating her with the great help of the local Fire Dept. We established bleeding control and finished packaging her in Spinal Precautions. She was following commands and maintaining her airway. We elected to "Load and Go", and deal with airway Enroute if necessary. We cleared the Scene and lifted just as two other Birds were landing in proximity for additional support. We had only been On-Scene for grand total of 16 minutes! Enroute, we placed IO access, gave fluids and analgesia, maintained bleeding control and continued to monitor her airway. She remained stable with surprisingly hyperdynamic vitals and the call went on without further drama. We did our turnover at the Trauma Center, and then we expeditiously loaded up and left to open another spot on the Helipad for incoming Birds.

The next morning, as we were wrapping up our shift, and doing our customary follow-up with the Facility Trauma Coordinator, we got an exciting piece of news!

It turns out, in addition to what we already knew, Grandma had a Stage 4 Liver Laceration which required immediate surgery. Grandma had survived the surgery and was stable in the SICU recovering. My Partner and I were stoked!

We were almost sidetracked a couple times by all the chaos. Yet the most time-sensitive and fragile Pt On-Scene was the LAST Pt we came across. I guess the take-home advice here is: Make sure when you are Triaging On-Scene- YOU DONT MISS GRANDMA!

CHAPTER 18 : FREEWAY LANDINGS

Freeway landings are very fun! My Father always calls it "Bringing In The Herd!", because of the dramatically charged spectacle it creates. Anyway, it's important to remember, depending on the freeway- You may or may not be blocking multiple traffic lanes in one or both directions of travel. Time is of the essence, as the local Highway Patrol Officers will be sure to remind you. So typically, you want to "Scoop and Run". If you must RSI On-Scene, then you are doing so in "A Particularly Expeditious Fashion".

*- Another important thing to keep in mind about being On-Scene (This goes for any Scene, but particularly closed freeway Scenes)- You are under observation by potentially hundreds of people and being recorded by at least dozens of them. So be very careful, even more careful than normal, about what you say and do while On-Scene. You are "Flying In and Saving The Day" according to every pair of eyes watching. Half the people watching are staring at us like we are Superheroes (Which we

are!). Look and act accordingly please. Also, if your Protocols require you to wear safety reflective vests (Or whatever) on freeway/roadway Scenes, you better wear them- Because you are going to be on at least a few internet postings by the end of the hour and on the Evening News. In the modern age there is nowhere to hide if you looked, acted, or performed stupidly! THE BEST STRATEGY IS TO ALWAYS BEHAVE AS THOUGH YOU ARE ON CAMERA. Because you probably are!

CHAPTER 19 : AIRWAY ARTISTRY & GOOD ADVICE

SCENARIO QUESTION: Do we RSI unstable Trauma Pts On-Scene or "Load and Go" and RSI Enroute to the Trauma Center?

SCENARIO ANSWER: SITUATION DICTATES! Discuss with your Partner and make a decision. QUICKLY.

*- This might mean loading up a deteriorating Pt in a hurry and "Securing The Airway" Enroute. It is certainly not ideal to RSI while In-Flight. I have done it a few different times and in a couple of different Bird configurations. They all went fine, crowded and chaotic, but successful on all occasions!

Performing RSI In-Flight is much easier if you have drilled this Procedure in your head and performed hands-on simulation training in your Bird.

- TIPS FOR SUCCESSFUL RSI:

- **PRE-OXYGENATE PROPERLY!** A mnemonic acronym I thought up is ENTAPS (Emergency Nurses Train And Practice Safely):

E- Elevate HOB ~30 Degrees (You lose lung volume lying flat!)

N- Nasal Cannula (High-Flow)

T- Two Thumbs Up Bagging

A- Alternate Airways (NPA's and having a "Plan B" (CRICH))

P- Peep

S- Suction

----

*- PUSH-DOSE PRESSORS:

Use them. Use them early. Use them often. Maintain Perfusion Pressure before and during RSI - Or all your meticulous RSI efforts will have been for nothing when your Pt codes mid-attempt.

----

*- Do mock In-Flight RSI training for each different Bird setup!

- DIRECT LARYNGOSCOPY (DL):

- Do Not Knock Out Teeth!

(But if you do, then at least have the courtesy to put them back in!)

- No DL on SMR/C-Spine Pts - DON'T HURT TRAUMA NECKS!

(This is one of the biggest reasons for "Video Laryngoscopy" (VL) in the first place!) Keep reading for a great RSI story!

*- When checking laryngoscope bulbs, leave on for at least 5 full seconds to ensure proper charge (And have spares of course, "Just In Case").

- Imagine you are intubating your loved one. BE GENTLE. Deliberate, but Smooth!

*- Magill Forceps are worth their weight in gold!!!

- VIDEO LARYNGOSCOPY (VL):

VL is the way of the future, be comfortable with it, and get used to it! There will definitely be times where some sort of equipment failure or weird situation will necessitate DL (Intense ambient brightness negates plasma screen; Battery depletion; Bloody or wet airway; etc.). The camera can't see through fluid. This means sometimes, even if you're pre-suctioning or continuously suctioning, you will still have a gooey wet airway. Once the camera is soaked, it's usually not an easy clean with BSI in place, and then you're going to need to switch to a DL approach. Some devices are geniously engineered to facilitate both VL and DL! These are awesome!

- BOUGIES:

Use Them routed through your ETT as a leading guidewire. Coil them with the curved contour of the ETT and with a little practice you can have incredible dexterity every bit as effective as with a rigid stylet.
The only people who do not like using them are old school old timers who are too proud, lazy, selfish, insecure, or ignorant to realize the Pt safety benefits and embrace a new technique.

SHAME ON THEM!

It gives you a bailout plan to secure the airway on the first attempt. If you cannot thread the tube, then bury the bougie and then slide the tube down- Done and Done!

Bougies are ingenious. Why would you not use them if able? End of discussion.

----

*- DO NOT FORGET TO CHECK THE BLOOD GLUCOSE LEVEL (BGL) FOR ANY ALTERED PT! Please do not be the complacent caregiver who just RSI'd an ALOC (Altered Level Of Consciousness) Pt- Only to find later during the Secondary Assessment the Glucose is 20!

- BREATH SOUNDS:

*- If uncertain about breath sounds: Always say "Diminished" or "Decreased" or an honestly blatant "Unable to Obtain". This shows an attempt to be "Intellectually honest" and gives the receiving Caregiver a need to reassess lung sounds properly. Do not lazily say lung sounds are "Clear" unless you are absolutely certain.

----

*- DO NOT EVER MISS A **TENSION PNEUMOTHORAX**!!! ANYTIME YOU HAVE A DETERIORATING PT AND YOU ARE NOT 100% POSITIVE WHY THEY ARE DETERIORATING = NEEDLE TIME!!!

- "TOMAHAWK" INTUBATION:

This is an "Advanced Technique" where you intubate someone from the front. This means passing the tube with your LT Hand and holding the Laryngoscope upside down with your RT Hand. Funky right!?! I know. It takes some practice. You need to be comfortable with this technique, because there are numerous situations where it is useful. A trapped Pt deteriorating during extrication and you must RSI them from the hood of the vehicle. Or perhaps you have a shotgun blast to the face you can't lay flat without drowning, so you sit them upright against the wall and RSI them. That's just a couple of examples. I'm sure you can think of plenty more. Try it on an intubation dummy sometime so you can add this to your RSI "Bag of Tricks".

- SURGICAL AIRWAYS:

As a former "Green Side" Platoon Corpsman, my answer to everything is "Crich 'Em!". That being said, you better be able to justify any Surgical Airway you place. Paradoxically, you need to RECOGNIZE EARLY when it's time to "Crich". DON'T SCREW AROUND! **"Make the Decision, then Make the Incision!"**. We are all going to have Pts die on us, BUT THEY BETTER DIE WITH A FREAKIN AIRWAY!!!

- KEEP YOUR PT SEDATED AND COMFORTABLE:

For your Intubated/Sedated Pts, attempt to raise their "Rousability Threshold" by utilizing "Stimuli-Reduction" tools. Earplugs and Blindfolds (If not contraindicated) are excellent tools for making your Pt's sedation more effective. This obviously helps keep them more "Comfortable and Ventilator Compliant". This will also decrease (To varying degrees) the sedation dosage requirements needed to achieve goals.

*- Obviously, this won't always be practical! If you have a 6-point restrained 300 lb belligerent drunk with a head injury whom you RSI'd On-Scene and they are violently rousing from the worn-off paralytic or follow-up sedation.....Then I know earplugs and blindfolds aren't going to do a bit of good! Stop being silly! The only things which will make a difference in this

case is high-dose sedation & rope! If "Operational Safety" is in question, "Physically Restrain" or re-paralyze as necessary to RAPIDLY achieve "Situational Control" and "Mission Safety". Follow your own company Protocols for "Combative Pt Management". You need to MEMORIZE these Protocols. It is very "Need to Know" information when you "Need to Know" it. Please be prepared!

- VENTILATORS AND VENTILATION STRATEGY:

This topic has already been covered in-depth by some of our brilliant Colleagues. So, I am referring you to them. Please read and enjoy Charlie Swearingen's, Eric Bauer's, and Dr William Owen's respective books, which are listed in the back of this Bible.

*- I do feel obligated to make a quick mention of the famous "D.O.P.E." mnemonic for Ventilator Troubleshooting:

D - Dislodged Tube

O - Obstruction

P - Pneumothorax

E - Equipment

KNOW THIS MNEMONIC WELL! IT SHOULD BE A CONSTANT MENTAL EXERCISE/REASSESSMENT TOOL FOR YOUR INTUBATED PTS.

- OXYGEN:

Put Oxygen on Every Pt!

(As appropriate obviously)

(Most Non-Respiratory Pts will be fine on a NC at 2 lpm)
I am sure a lot of RT's and Pulmonologists would have much more complicated ways of saying the following bit, but I'm going to do us a favor and speak plainly.

- Keep the SPO2 between 94% - 99%. This will ensure you are in an appropriate range.
- We avoid 100% SPO2 because 100% could actually be 200% or 300% or more!
(Remember during your Pathophysiology lectures in Nursing School they discussed potential complications from Hyperoxia? No? Well then look it up again!)
- There are many benefits of Oxygen application in Non-Pulmonary Pts. O2 helps combat the effects of nausea, motion sickness, and flicker vertigo. There is also a psychosomatic element worth noting.
- O2 will also preemptively treat the Pt's inevitable desaturation if you are going high up in altitude (Pop Quiz: Which Gas Law is this? You're going to need to know!)

- USE YOUR SUCTION!:

Pts are secured tightly (Hopefully), and it can be difficult for them to clear secretions. So help them out with oral suction! These Pts might even be able to self-suction, making everybody's day easier.

- GIVE ANTIEMETICS before ANY opiates, and IV PUSH OPIATES SLOWLY! Just trust me. Puking makes everything worse for everyone! Especially for your spine-boarded Pts. This is a lesson you don't need to learn firsthand!

- VFIB WITH SEVERE HYPOTHERMIA ISN'T A MYTH!:

That's right folks, be ready for it! If you incidentally shake, rattle, or roll your severely hypothermic Pt, then you are consequently going to most likely be doing ACLS. Do what you can to minimize bumps and aggressive movements.

- VENTRIC DRAIN TIP!:

Fortunately my Partner and I recognized this issue ahead of time, and we were ready for it, but I want to make a quick mention of a unique potential problem with Ventric drainage systems and Transport. The Pt will most likely end up, however briefly, in a steep head-up or head-down angle during RW or FW Aircraft sled onloading Procedures or takeoff/landing. This angle will vary greatly from Aircraft to Aircraft. Some will have front loading where you go feet first. Some rear loading, where you go head first, etc. Any time the Pt's head is higher than the ventric drain, excessive drainage can rapidly occur. Be sure to temporarily and briefly clamp the drain in these situations, to avoid excessive CSF drainage THIS IS ESPECIALLY RELEVANT DURING TAKEOFF IN A JET - Where the entire Bird comes screaming off the ground at very exciting bank angles! People don't realize these Jets can go upwards of 550 mph! When they take off, they REALLY take off!!! (But Helicopters are still way cooler!)

*- DO NOT FORGET TO UNCLAMP THE VENTRIC DRAIN AND "ZERO" AT THE APPROPRIATE LEVEL ONCE THE INTENSE-ANGLE CHANGING EVENT IS OVER! Failure to do this WILL potentially result in further Brain damage secondary to ever-increasing ICP during Transport.

- WAIT TIL WE ARE AIRBORNE PLEASE!:

It is a great idea, whenever possible, to have your Ground Ambulance standby and wait until you are airborne. Just in case a WCS happens between closing those doors and takeoff..... It could be a change in Pt status; A mechanical issue; A severely prolonged runway wait time- Who knows?!?
I realize this won't always be possible. Ground Ambulances usually have places to go, people to see, and things to eat- But try to keep it in mind as an Intelligent Strategy!

CHAPTER 20 : HOW WE SAVED A LIFE

A while back, we were landing on a busy, closed-down desert freeway for a mess of an MVC. We didn't have much Pt info yet, but while we were circling above doing our landing Procedures, we could see a large crash debris field and the remaining sliver from the front driver's side of a silver sedan. There was an 18-wheeler nearby with damage and debris as well, so we were getting the idea- Somebody had attempted to pass the truck, hadn't made it, and was run over by the giant tractor trailer. Judging from the severity of vehicular damage, it was doubtful anyone in the sedan survived. There was a Ground Ambulance in the middle of the road near where we were going to be setting down, we presumed our Pt was inside. We landed on the closed down freeway, the Pilot kept the Bird running, and we went to evaluate what was in the back of the Ambulance. We opened the side door to find blood dripping out around the frame..........

......always a great sign. The Pt was a young woman, about 20 yrs old, and weighing approx 60kg. There was blood everywhere, and a Firefighter was attempting to wrap the Pt's head. I looked over and saw she had been partially scalped, but her skull appeared otherwise intact. She was in full

Spinal Precautions. She was awake, but very lethargic and confused with delayed response. Despite the blood loss, she was hemo-dynamically stable and oxygenating well. While there were no other "Obvious Life-Threatening Injuries" to speak of; My Partner and I discussed how her neck was probably "Mangled" pretty good by the scalping mechanism and the obvious severity of the MVC. At this point, my Partner and I instantly agreed the Pt needed to be RSI'd. We dove into our practiced routine of quickly setting up equipment, drawing up medications, pre-oxygenating, etc. I was going to be performing the intubation on this call (My Partner and I took turns, and I was up to bat!). Our company had recently switched to a new cutting edge VL setup, which we were mandated to use as our primary laryngoscope. I had been practicing with the new device and adored it! It makes great sense for use on Trauma Pts because there is no aggressive neck manipulation. We went through the "RSI Checklist" and smoothly placed the tube on the first attempt. We finished packaging, loaded up, and made time for the Trauma Center. We completed turnover, high-fived each other, and headed back to Base. Just another call. Our initial "End of Shift" follow up with the Trauma Center confirmed she had survived and was stable. Good stuff!

Two months later I received a phone call while I was on shift at the Base. It was my Partner from the call, he said "Hey Rob-Check your work email! Good job Partner! Congrats!". Unsure what to expect, I anxiously opened the file and there was a letter from a Case Manager at a Rehab Facility. The letter informed us our Pt's injuries included multiple unstable Cervical Fractures of C-3 through C-7! The letter also said our Pt was in "Halo" neck brace, was WALKING, and wanted to meet the Ground and Flight Crews who saved her life! Wow. My immediate first thought was: IF I WOULD HAVE BROKEN PROTOCOL AND GONE DL FOR THE INTUBATION, I WOULD HAVE CERTAINLY MADE HER A QUADRIPLEGIC! Attached was a picture of our Pt, walking at the Rehab Facility and waving with an ear to ear grin. With admittedly moist eyes, I reflected on how big a "Win" this was. "Happily Everafter" does not happen every day in FlightWorld. This was a perfect example of how modern technology, proper equipment selection, and up-to-date technique saved a young woman's quality of life! THIS IS WHY WE DO THIS, AND WHY WE ATTEMPT TO DO IT AS PERFECTLY AS POSSIBLE!

CHAPTER 21 : KETAMINE

This is not a textbook or a research paper. So, I am going to say a couple things about Ketamine and then immediately tell you to go online and research this Wonder Drug!

Ketamine got a bad rap for years because it was associated with some negative results in a study about increased ICP. Those results have since been re-evaluated and tossed out by Prevailing Research and Evidence Based Practice. Ketamine is the "New Generation's" RSI Sedation Induction Agent of choice and is included in most Flight Protocols Nationwide! Why is this so important and awesome? Why do I care?

BECAUSE IT IS A SEDATIVE THAT SUPPORTS SYMPATHETIC TONE AND DOESN'T HURT YOUR BLOOD PRESSURE!

This sounds too good to be true! Are you kidding me?!? Incredible! The potential usefulness of a Wonder Drug like this is invaluable! Especially in unstable Trauma Pts! Just imagine how much easier life would be without the potential for "Hypotensive Complications" from your Induction Sedative. Ketamine gives an extra "Sympathetic Tone Buffer" every time you RSI a fragile/borderline hemodynamically unstable Pt.

Ketamine is Revolutionary! - And while research is ongoing, I am very glad the National EMS and HEMS Community has embraced this Wonder Drug!

*- Ketamine is obviously not the RSI Sedation Induction Agent of choice in the presence of Severe HTN. The Increased Sympathetic Tone will only make combating HTN more difficult (Duh!). If you are in a Hypertensive Crisis, then Ketamine is not the preferred drug anyway, since other sedative choices will additionally combat HTN.

*- This section is only discussing Ketamine as a Sedative Agent! Ketamine is also an Analgesic, but this is a very different (However Fun!) conversation for another time.

CHAPTER 22 : A PRESSOR PRIMER

- "VASO" PRESSOR USE WITH SEDATION:

*- This is assuming NORMOvolemia! If your Pt is HYPOvolemic, then give volume per Protocol before jumping straight to a pressor. Or do both to be safe and prevent deterioration! Then re-evaluate the need for a continuous pressor after bolusing some fluid. THIS IS CALLED "BEING PROACTIVE INSTEAD OF REACTIVE"! THIS IS - **"THE WAY OF THE FLIGHT KNIGHT"**.

SCENARIO: Here is an all-too-common situation you encounter regularly in the IFT realm. You encounter your intubated Pt resting in bed, in the dark, with minimal stimuli and restraints applied. Some combination of low-dose analgesia and sedation is most likely in use. This Pt is wide awake, bucking the tube, and in obvious discomfort. Their SBP is in the low 90's or worse.

What do you do? This is Flight Knight 101 stuff! The answer is YOU START A PRESSOR! An "Alpha-effect" pressor would be ideal in this case- Unless advanced CHF complications call for more intense "Beta-effect" pressors, or a combination of a "Beta" pressor and "SVR Reduction" drug combo. This will protect your Pt's perfusion while allowing you to titrate up your sedation to provide for appropriate Pt comfort! This seems like common sense right?!? EVIDENTLY NOT!

Some of you still haven't become comfortable enough with pressor calculations or gtt management. As a result of this ignorance, your Pt has to be "Near Death" before you will use a pressor. **You don't have to wait until your Pt is "In extremis" to use pressors. An elite Flight Knight will routinely use a pressor to avoid being "In extremis" in the first place!**

There is another issue to discuss here- We must address Pt comfort more appropriately! I have seen colleagues continue restraints; Leave the inadequately sedated Pt bucking the tube and flopping like a fish; Then start an hour-long Transport across town. FOR SHAME!

"PRESSORS PREVENT STRESSORS"

There is an old Transport joke- "If your intubated Pt remembers you, you suck!".

*- PUSH-DOSE PRESSORS:

Use them. Use them early. Use them often. The End.

CHAPTER 23 : GOING THE EXTRA MILE

*- These suggestions will help bridge the gap between being a "Great Clinician" and being a "Great Caregiver".

Outside of "Saving Lives" and "Being Awesome Clinically", there are many small things we can do to make our Pt's Transport better and the overall situation more optimal.

- Follow up with drop-off facilities for Pt status.

- Thank collaborating agencies post-call. Keep an email template ready to fill out and send. This goodwill helps build better Community Resources and relationships. These agencies are the one's calling us! We want to be nice to them!

- Take family contact info On-Scene to follow-up with status after turnover at receiving facility (If the situation allows- Do Not significantly delay Transport!).

- Keep a spare pair of dark sunglasses in the Helicopter to put on Pts to reduce "Flicker Vertigo". (Not kidding)

- Inflatable head/neck pillows. These are super cheap to bulk-buy online and offer on every Flight (Where SMR is not already in place, of course!).

- Have a portable phone charging source with a couple adapter options for your conscious and alert Pts. Their phone is their only lifeline to normalcy at this moment, and of course their battery will be nearly dead, causing terrible anxiety. I know it sounds silly, but just think about the last time you were without a charger and your phone died. Or the last time your phone broke, and you were without for a few hours while you went to the store for a replacement or whatever...... IT'S AWEFUL RIGHT?!? We can avoid this additional stressor by simply having a charger for them.

- RECEIVING/GIVING A CALM TURNOVER AND SMOOTH ONLOAD/OFFLOAD PACKAGING:

*- **THE ART OF THE "SLOW ROLL"** - Another one of my early mentors once approached me after a call and told me I needed to slow down and be calmer. He said my intensity On-Scene or At Bedside was causing stress without me even realizing it. Here I am, thinking I am controlling the situation and being appropriately assertive to achieve efficient results. When in actuality, I was a visibly tense bundle of dynamite and was creating stress by my very demeanor. He told me I needed to SLOW ROLL my calls. This obviously does not mean being slow, but rather CALM. Assertive but Relaxed. Efficient yet Graceful. Proud but Humble. This is not as easy as it sounds. I struggled with it for years, in fact, I STILL struggle. But it can be done! I've done it. Everything is smoother, your colleagues are nicer, the Pt is calmer........ SLOW ROLL!
SLOW IS SMOOTH and SMOOTH IS FAST.

----

*- DO NOT ROLL YOUR EYES OR SIGH DURING REPORT! JUST DONT! Take this one from me. Just smile, nod, and get out drama free! We Nurses are a vindictive and moody bunch. We will absolutely call your company and get you written up for rudeness. Ask me how I know!

We must remind ourselves continuously: These Pts, Hospital Staff, and Ground Crews Are Our Customers!

----

*- Anybody can become a Flight Nurse if they want it bad enough, but **"The Art Is In The Perfection"**.

There are millions of Nurses in the USA and many millions more all over the World. What makes you special? How are going to stand out? What are you going to stand for? How are you going to be remembered? Ask yourself these questions. Then change the world for the better with your answers!

PART IV - GROUNDWORLD & GEAR GUIDELINES

CHAPTER 24 : GROUNDWORLD & CCT

- AMBULANCE DRIVING SAFETY TIPS:

- Slow Down!!!

- Decrease speed before the turn! Before the wheel turns the tires, the Ambulance needs to have slowed down already, or you are launching everyone in the back across the rig. GroundWorld Physics 101! Decrease speed so you need to accelerate to complete a turn- Not slow down in the middle of a turn because you are already going too fast!

- INCREASE FOLLOWING DISTANCE!

Whatever you think a good following distance is -
DOUBLE IT!!!
(and TRIPLE it if raining!)

*- It's hard to get in a front-end collision if there's nothing in front of you!

- CHECK YOUR RIG AT BEGINNING OF EVERY SHIFT:

- Eyeball the tires.

- Check Lights & Sirens

- Check the fuel and oil levels.

- Med Bag Inventory.

- Is O2 tank topped off?

- Does inverter turn on and electrical outlets work?

- Does the suction unit turn on and have adequate pressure?

- Is VHF/UHF Radio turning on and functioning?

- Do we have all our Bags? (Do **"Number Count"**!)

- Do we have an OB kit?

- Do we have blankets?

and ANYTHING else you can think of.

- SEATBELTS AND "THE HIPPOCRATIC HYPOCRITE":

We all know we should wear a seatbelt in the back of the rigs, but rarely do we actually do it. Well, if you have "Medic Catcher" webbing nets in your rig, then I guess you can justify being unbelted a little bit..... but here's the plain truth:

If the driver locks up the breaks or worse- Hits something or gets hit by someone- You are going flying into whatever jagged surfaces at whatever body smashing speeds the Laws of Physics dictate.

That said, do I always wear a seatbelt?

My Official Answer: "Of course! Every time, all the time, without fail, ever!".

My Honest Answer: "No, of course not, but I really should!". **It's a preventable and stupid way to die.**

- "A-BAG" (Ground CCT Ambulance Gear Bag):

Within reason, gear weight doesn't matter in GroundWorld. My "A-Bag" is loaded to the gills with all sorts of eccentric equipment/gear I do not carry in FlightWorld. Because in FlightWorld, my personal carry-on "H-Bag" (Helicopter gear bag) and my "J-Bag" (Jet/Fixed Wing bag) are necessarily weight and space limited. This means I have all sorts of "Questionably Excessive" "WCS-Resolving" gizmos, doodads, thingamabobs, and gadgets in my A-Bag. I jokingly refer to my A-Bag as "Twenty pounds of **'Don't worry, I've got this!'**".

- TARMAC TURNOVER:

There have been occasions where I have performed pickups and handoffs at International Airports; On the tarmac with other Flight Crews or Ground Transport Crews. In a perfect FlightWorld, there would be a "Continuum of Transport Care", and I would accompany the Pt to their final destination. However, you will encounter all sorts of odd, random, annoyingly spontaneous, and potentially disruptive situations requiring an out-of-facility turnover of Pt care. In this case, it's obviously most important to keep the Pt safe and comfortable from the elements.

Then special attention must be applied to giving an adequate and appropriate, yet expediently "On-the-go" report to the new Caregivers. Along with the Chart, Meds, Belongings, Chihuahua (Yes, that happened!), etc. Oh, and all this will hopefully be in your native language, English in my case. There might be significant language barriers. Do the best you can. Use a multilingual type translation app for text conversing. Also be sure to utilize any translation service your company might provide. You are responsible for giving a thorough and appropriate turnover for your Pt. Do not overlook this very crucial and important part of the job. Do what you must do to communicate properly. Then meticulously document it!

- GROUND CCT "BORDERLAND" PICKUPS:

 I have done much of my Ground Ambulance CCT work in Southern California. This means I've had many interesting "Border Pickups". These pickups almost always occur in a holding area at the U.S-Mexico Border called "Secondary". This is a football field sized parking lot filled with vehicles requiring additional "Attention". Most often it's a document issue, random license check, inspection, etc. It's a chaotic place. This is essentially "Neutral Ground" where U.S.

Ground Ambulances meet Mexican Ground Ambulances.

 I've had many "Screwball Secondary" Border Pickup Scenarios which were "Character Building" (To say the least!).
Including:
- On MULTIPLE occasions, encountering decompensated, "In-extremis" Pts which were "Fine Five Minutes Ago" (Estaban Bien Hace Cinco Minutos). Which we then would begin salvaging and perform a "Scoop and Grab" outta there!
- Having an awake, tied down, gagging intubated Pt because the Mexican "EMTs" didn't have an IV pump to continue the Pt's sedation gtt.
- Having family members detained for document issues and becoming hysterical and combative with Border Patrol because we must continue transporting without them.
- Getting reprimanded for allowing foreign fruits and vegetables into the Country because we didn't search our Pt's luggage (Gimme a break.....).
- And my personal favorite, the time I was nearly charged for "Human Trafficking"! Border Patrol Agents followed our rig to the Hospital because THEY loaded up a Ridealong family member whom (Unbeknownst to me) hadn't had their documents examined yet. I explained the situation and how we

were in no way at fault, but they were still really mad! I was getting phone calls from Border Patrol Case Agents and Supervisors for a month afterwards............... Sheesh. Anyway, just another day in "Secondary".

I suppose the takeaway lesson here is to be ready! Because anything can, and probably will, happen down in "BorderLand"!

CHAPTER 25 : PERSONAL & SURVIVAL GEAR

*- Gear is a very personal thing. You will have a fun time undergoing "R&D" for your own setup. I am going to outline some general recommendations, guidelines, and tips for equipment and related features.

Every "Gear Nerd" has their own "Must have" and "Can't live without" items they will rave about. I recommend listening to people's recommendations when they are passionate about a piece of equipment. Odds are if somebody is super excited to unselfishly advertise for a specific product, it is probably awesome! Check it out so you don't miss out!

- PERSONAL FLIGHT GEAR:

There are only a few general rules about Personal Flight Gear:

#1: Gear should be relatively lightweight and compact.

#2: Gear needs to be durable, reliable, and preferably multi-purpose.

#3: Gear needs to look like something a vigilante Superhero would carry and use!

Many employers will have strict equipment and uniform regulations for personal suit and equipment configuring. Some places are more relaxed and allow their employees to self-outfit as they desire.

Who knows where you will end up and what the Protocols will be, but you want to strike a balance between being adequately prepared and not being weighted down with stuff you never use. More is not always better, sometimes more is just more. That being said, always have more than less. Always be overprepared and never underprepared.

Attempt to be practical when loading up your pockets/ vest/ pouches/ "Chocket" (Chest-pocket harness setup)/ etc. Because you don't want to be the awkward goofy stereotypical "Ricky-Rescue" weirdo who has all the wrong priority gear. You shouldn't have a frying pan in your Flight Gear....... for example. (An espresso machine however..........)

----

*- ON-PERSON, IN-FLIGHTSUIT SURVIVAL GEAR:

- This is about carrying a few special survival items in your Flightsuit pockets to have in the event of surviving a crash and being stranded for a potentially lengthy period of time- While potentially being significantly injured and in shock over the loss of your fellow Flight Crewmembers/Pt. It's a pretty short list, but I want to "Plant the seed" and prepare you for the WCS:

- Reflective Survival Blanket

- Bilateral Blades (Ambidextrous knife access)

- An effectively intense Tourniquet (Pre-configured for self-application)

- 14ga Decompression Needle (For self)

- Waterproof matches

- Whistle

- Saint Bernard Dog with barrel of brandy around its neck.

- A Homing Pigeon or a Raven (Way cooler) for carrying news of your survival to rescuers.

- Compact/Portable Cellphone Charger device to keep your phones GPS transmitting or signal light strobe ready to use to attract Rescuers. You also MIGHT have a decent phone signal and can call your dispatch with coordinates for RESCUE, or your loved ones to say **GOODBYE.**

----

*- I know this is morbid stuff. At some point in your Career it WILL happen to you or someone you know. Guaranteed.

I have flown with several Crash Survivors and slept in the "Beds of The Dead". I once floated to a Base to cover a shift after they had a fatal crash which killed the Pilot and Nurse. I closed the door to the Nurses' bedroom to lay down and on the back of the door I saw a typical crayon scribble drawing of a house, family and dog. Across the top were the words "Love You Daddy". The dead Nurses' Child had drawn it the week before. I wept. There are many more tragic stories like this one, but they don't need to be told here. Just make sure you truly understand the huge responsibility you accept "SO OTHERS MAY LIVE".

CHAPTER 26 : SPECIFIC GEAR ITEMS & FEATURES

- TRAUMA SHEARS:

They are an important and necessary tool for every Healthcare Provider! You can carry a generic cheap pair and call it a day....OR- You can be awesome and have a tactical and envy inducing set of intense trauma shears! Your choice, and it depends on the environment and the rest of your gear setup. On my person, I usually carry a blacked-out pair of the medium sized surgical shears with a couple hemostats (Serrated and Non-serrated). I bulk buy these smaller shears because quite often On-Scene you will share them and lose them. I also carry more "Heavy Duty" tactical shears in a sheath on the strap of my Personal Flight Bag. I like placing an aftermarket screw-on reverse-direction clothes/seat belt-cutter device which affixes to the underside of the lower handle. There are custom holster models made to accommodate these. Quite often these add-on pieces will also have an O2 wrench as well, which is nice. I am sure there are plenty of other cool and inventive designs out there, the best idea is to go online and go hunting!

- POCKETKNIVES:

Personal carry pocketknives need to be practically sized (2-3"
blade is fine). Remember, we want a compact blade to have on
our Flightsuit. This knife is not meant for Dragon-Slaying or
Crocodile-Wrangling. Those types of knives are fine for
wherever else in life, but here we are talking about "On-Person"
compact/semi compact "Tactical and Practical" daily use blades.

*- An obvious, yet "Painful to learn the hard way" tip about
pocket knife safety: When a pocketknife is in your pocket, the
closed blade needs to be positioned in the REAR lining of the
pocket. So if you accidentally "Assist open" your knife, or reach
into your pocket awkwardly to grab something else- You don't
slice your hand open or catch it on the blade. If the unfolding
blade is set into the REAR seam of the respective pocket, the
blade should be out of the way. A lot of knives might not be
setup ideally for left or right dominant pocket practicality in
this sense. Keep this in mind, and please be careful! This
technique should also ensure accidentally-opened blades are
always pointed laterally away from your genital regions.
(Ouch!!! I don't even want to think about it, PLEASE BE
CAREFUL!)

- MULTITOOLS (The "Don't Worry, I Got This!" Stick):

You are going to need one of these! You do not know what for- This is the whole point! But you are definitely going to need one sooner or later, so you better have one! They need to have a very capable plier set, liner-locking attachment blades, seatbelt/ clothing cutter, screwdrivers, O2 wrench, etc. They need to have a pocket ready side clip- You (Generally) do not wear a belt with a Flightsuit, so finding a practical and easily accessible pouch attachment location isn't going to be ideal. You want to keep this multitool tucked into your Flightsuit pocket on the OPPOSITE side of your pocket knife pocket. This way you can ambidextrously get to a blade quickly in the event of WCS.

- HEADLAMP FLASHLIGHTS (Or "Hang Around Neck" Lamps)(Separate from "Helmet Mounted" options):

There are a variety of cool options out there but essentially, they need to be relatively compact, lightweight, durable, and powerful. I prefer lights that take batteries instead of a charge, because I can always replace/swap out disposable or rechargeable batteries faster than I can charge a device (Duh). Your light also needs a red, blue, or green "Nightlight" option. Because these colors do not destroy anyone's night vision! A slide on/off button is nice. White light to one direction, "Nightlight" to the other. Some models even have a built-in external slide down lense which covers the light.

*- The models to avoid are where a single click button rotates thru the light types. This is obviously STUPID because what is the point of switching to the "Nightlight" option if you must destroy your night vision first by click-cycling thru white light options? Right!?! Drives me crazy!

*- DO NOT FORGET SPARE AA's AND AAA's FOR YOUR FLASHLIGHTS!

(Or whatever spare batteries you might need)

- KNOT TYING:

This knowledge is very useful and important, but do not get carried away. A few simple knots will cover your needs for most situations. I personally suggest first learning how to use a "Square Knot", "Sailor's Hitch", and "Figure Eight".

Also, you should intimately know how to rapidly and blindfolded tie a "Self-Bowline" and a "Single Hand Bowline" for Hoist Rescue (Ambidextrously, of course. Unless your Crystal Ball tells you in advance which arm you are going to break).

These are the "Bare-bones" knots you must know and know in both single and double forms (One or two strand) with reinforcement (Typically repetitive "Overhand" type simple knots until your OCD is satisfied).

See? That's not too bad. Half dozen knots or so and you're a Tactical Guru!

- CARABINERS:

"I'm a big enthusiast for Things that connect Things to other Things!"

There are many cool tactical carabiner and connector options nowadays! One can get dizzy with choices! Find cool load-bearing options and keep them handy! You will find no shortage of daily uses for the these invaluable "Extra Hand" devices.

Small and medium carabiners are ideal for grouping and organizing multiple gtt bags/bottles/syringes for Transport. This keeps lines organized for a more streamlined and tidier offload/handoff.

*- I know some of you are thinking: We never Transport glass! Don't we always draw up glass bottle contents in syringes? While I agree this is a good practice (Especially if you want all the air out of the system.) - A lot of places use foam rubber sleeves for glass bottles which makes them safer and more practical.

- STETHOSCOPES:

Personally, I am half-deaf (From a lifetime of Loud Guitar Playing and Gunfire), so I more or less carry a stethoscope for "Totemistic" and "Professional Accountability" purposes.

This actually is mostly fine in FlightWorld, because stethoscopes are USELESS in a running Helicopter. Sure, I keep one coiled in the pant leg pocket of my Flightsuit to listen On-Scene or At Bedside during an IFT. But due to the extremely heightened assessment skills of the elite Flight Knight- Stethoscopes are a luxury. They aren't going to tell you anything Critical that a keen eye and a good set of Vital Signs (Including ETCO2) won't.

- "BUILDING A STETHOSCOPE":
I am going to vaguely explain how someone might possibly acquire an expensive stethoscope "Replica" which is high quality and a fraction the cost. Go online for "Replacement" tubing and "Replica" stethoscope heads for ANY highspeed brand (Wink). You will find a decently priced SINGLE-DIAPHRAGM "Cardiac-Specific" head for cheap. Then you can buy the THICK SINGLE TUBE quality replica/replacement tubing for any color desired (I recommend black or radical

neon!). You have just separately pieced together a VERY quality stethoscope for ~$50 that list prices for ~$200. Look online, BE CLEVER, and you will see what I am talking about! Your welcome!

- LIP BALM/MENTHOL NASAL INHALER (Homemade Dual-Tool):

You are going to want to make one of these custom devices, and it is silly how easy it is. All you do is get a stick of your favorite spf rated lip balm and one of those menthol nasal inhaler sticks (They are the same size as the lip balm tube). Tape them together, slightly off centered and with the opening ends facing opposite sides. These two devices, separately and in-tandem, can make a world of difference in your mood. Especially when you are in a situation where life sucks and you are in 130-degree desert temps. A little bit of lip balm and a few deep nostril inhales of cool refreshing menthol will make you feel 100 times better. No joke. Take my word for it!

- STRAWS (For IFT use only):

In the emergent and crazy settings of FlightWorld or GroundWorld- Sometimes we overlook seemingly trivial items worth their weight in gold. Straws are one of these awesome items! Quite often, especially on International trips, you are going to be with a Pt who is not NPO and can self-feed and drink. Straws keep you and the Pt dry. It is hard to drink liquids when you're unable to sit up higher than 30-45 degrees and you can't lean forward properly due to safety restraints. It sounds silly, but trust me- It makes a world of difference and helps prevent choking and potential aspiration!

- NO PEPPER-SPRAY DEVICES!
*- THIS GOES FOR EVERYONE- Pt, Crew, Ridealongs, and ESPECIALLY Law Enforcement Ridealongs.

In the event of accidental discharge, you don't want your half-blinded Pilot performing an Emergency Landing because a pepper-spray device went off in the cabin.

- SNACKS AND NUTRITION (On The Go):

- Glucose Tabs! They are one of most important items you can carry! They will instantly improve your focus and mood!

- Protein bars which are chewy but dry and melt proof (No chocolate or peanut butter coatings, they will be a huge mess).

- Assorted flavor bags of peanuts or cashews.

- Assorted beef or turkey meat snack sticks or jerky.

- Non-melting candy of any favored variety.

- Chips and crackers (Although they are fragile and chip bags might pop in Flight) (POP QUIZ: WHAT GAS LAW IS THIS?).

- Water flavoring liquid or drink powders.

- Anything else small and hearty you can think of.

*- Please note the aforementioned items are "On the Go" food items and are not meant to be a balanced nutritional diet (Duh). When you are back at Base or at an FBO with time to spare, you need to eat Fruits, Vegetables, and Proteins!

- WATER AND HYDRATION:

- Have a decent sized (1.5 - 2 ltr) "Personal Water Source" (In addition to the "Crew Supply"). This source needs to be a padded and pliable water bladder variant, so it can fit in tight spaces as necessary.

- Straw-hose accessed hydration bags and their fabric carriers are ideal. The straw allows you to drink without getting soaking wet (It can be quite challenging drinking from a large lid water bottle with your Flight helmet on!)(Especially in a low-ceiling Helicopter design!)

*- Straw-tubing also allows you to access your water source discreetly without letting your Pt see it. Because I guarantee your Trauma, Cardiac, Neuro or Surgical Pt is very thirsty and most likely NPO. So we don't want to make them think about it. Out of sight, Out of mind! It's a simple, practical courtesy.

- Self-Hydration:
If you think you are drinking enough water, then you are WRONG! Drink More Water! Take it from the former "Greenside" Platoon Corpsman: While operating in extreme

temperatures, hot or cold- You cannot possibly drink enough water! When my Marines and I would be out in various deserts around the World doing "Our thing", I was constantly proselytizing the "Gospel of Hydration"! Quite often, I would pass out dry peppers to people to put in their mouths and chew on, because the subsequent burning and pain would force the individual to drink a ton of water- Regardless of how hot and disgusting the ambient temperature had made it. Because let's face it- Sometimes when you are in extreme elements, you do not even realize you are dehydrated until you are WAY dehydrated. By then you are a Heat Exhaustion/Heat Stroke candidate, and this takes an "Able Body Off A Working Rifle", which is obviously unacceptable.

*- I realize some of you are thinking, "Why not just drink cold water and stay hydrated? What's the big deal?" -
What do think this is?!? Some 5-star resort in Palm Springs with poolside service? No! I am talking about having to drink copious amounts of warm/hot gross ambiently temperatured water while working/operating in "Extreme Desert Conditions". Because you have no choice- It's lots of disgusting water or Heat Stroke!

- THE ARCTIC SUCKS! BRING A JACKET!:

Pack and take a warm outer layer clothing article with you, I have had several different experiences where we do a December pick up in Mexico or Central America at a balmy 80 degrees F and then Transport them to the Canadian Arctic where it is -60 degrees F with wind chill blasting like crazy! That is a 140 degree ambient temperature difference between pickup and drop-off! Absolutely Insane! I have never been so cold, I didn't even know it could get that cold! Wow!

So yeah..... Pack a compact/lightweight yet intensely warm jacket with a hood option. Also bring a warm hat, a neck or face wrap or ski-mask, and gloves. (For real- Being Cold Sucks!)

----

*- KEEP A PAIR OF PROTECTIVE TEXTURED GLOVES FOR TRACTION WITH HEAVY LIFTING/LOADING
(Especially relevant for FW Flights)

- BOOTS:

- As lightweight and streamlined as feasibly possible, while still offering a decent amount of high ankle support/ protection. There are lots of designs with fabric to leather ratios lighter in weight than bulky all-leather models.

- Protected toes (Composite toes are lighter than metal).

- Easy on/off accessibility (Side zip is a great option, or there are aftermarket front lace-to-zipper conversion devices which work just as well).

- Some form of quality gel footpad insert is a must. If your feet hurt after a long shift, this will make a world of difference! Your feet, knees, even your lower back will feel better! You should feel like you are walking on a cloud! These should be changed a couple times annually for best results.

- Vented options for boots are going to vary depending upon your main operating area. If you are in water up to your ankles daily, then low or side vented boots are a bad choice, whereas in the desert they are perfect! A lot of providers have separate seasonal boot options they prefer.

- Ultimately you are going to be spending a lot of time in these boots. You should genuinely like your boots and like to tell people how comfortable and awesome they are. This is valuable advice which might help a Colleague.

- HELMET SETUP AND ACCESSORIES:

The most important thing to remember about helmet accessories is to keep them super lightweight! Your neck and shoulders are already under constant strain from wearing your helmet for hours at a time. Especially at night with NVG's and the battery pack/additional counterweight. Cool accessories include:

- Mounting rails
- Push-button rotatable lights
- Dual Day and Night slide-down visors (Assorted colors available!)
- Lip-lights
- Flex-boom
- Noise cancelling system
- Stickers (YAY! I LOVE STICKERS! But PLEASE keep them appropriate for work! No WW2 Bomber Pinups!)
- NVG Counterweight/Battery Pack Mounting "Touch Fastener" Patch:

Most Experienced Flight Crewmembers mount a (Larger than necessary) "Touch Fastener" patch on the back of their helmets. Then they can stick their head to pre-existing gear mounting material on the wall. This keeps them upright while taking the load off their neck. It sounds silly, but just wait. This is especially helpful for very rural Bases with long Flight times.

- PERSONAL PHONE APPS YOU NEED:

- Dosage calc app.

- Second dosage calc app.

- An elite and comprehensive Critical Care app.

- A Pediatric Specific Critical Care app.

- Radio scanner app.

- O2 Tank Duration Calculator app.

- Multilingual conversational translation app or website.

- Your companies' Protocols bookmarked for easy access.

CHAPTER 27 : "OTHER" IMPORTANT GEAR ITEMS

*- "Shepherd's Crook" style Self-Massage Stick: A "MUST HAVE" back at Base.

Trust me, if you have never used one to loosen up your traps and massage around your scapulae, then you are missing out! Get one, use it regularly, and I guarantee you will feel less tight and tense, both physically and emotionally. There is almost nothing better than busting up deep tissue knots for helping your body relax! Especially your lateral neck muscle groups from supporting your helmet-heavy head.

- LIP BALM to apply PRN to provide proper mask-fit air seal for beards/facial hair. (Also great for Scuba Diving with a beard, but this is not very relevant here)

- PERSONAL MEDS: Glucose tabs, hydrocortisone cream, antibiotic ointment, nsaids, anti-emetics, antacids, etc.

- LADIES: Bring tampons, uti symptom relievers, nsaids, and whatever other special consideration items you might need.

- LBRT: A Length Based Resuscitation Tape is a mandatory "On-person" item. (Remember when we were talking about "Keeping away the Voodoo" with the OB Kit? Same thing here. Just keep one on you, this way you know you always have one.)

- Small Packet of Baby Wipes: Don't judge me! They keep your face, neck, ears, and whatever else clean and refreshed. You will be glad you have them!

- Large and Small Tampons for Bullet holes. (NOT KIDDING)

AFTERWORD and ADIEU

- EVERYTHING DOES NOT HAPPEN FOR A REASON!

Intelligent, self-respecting people need to stop saying otherwise. I mean, sure- You can derive a Scientific explanation of events to describe something which has occurred, whatever it may be. The Pt died because their head was injured while they were not wearing a helmet; You had an unplanned Pregnancy because you failed to properly utilize birth-control methods; You got or spread the Flu because you failed to Vaccinate; etc.

But to seriously suggest "Everything happens according to a plan" or to explain away endless mass destruction, tragedy, genocide, and pitiless suffering as "Part of god's plan" is intellectual suicide. It is mentally lazy and morally reprehensible to brush off tragedy as the workings of a completely intangible yet supposedly omnipotent entity. **All causes are local. Always!**

Everything in the Universe obeys a complex series of Mechanical/Physical Laws. To suggest these ever-present "Rules of Existence" are temporarily suspended for the particular benefit of an individual or group is silly nonsense.

There are Billions and Billions of People on this Beautiful Blue Planet, and we are all spinning through Space together for the entire term of our short lives. These facts should not depress you or make you feel small. These facts should inspire and empower you to look around the World and see the many ways you can make a "Positive Impact" with your existence.

If there is a "Greater Purpose to Life", it MUST be to "Serve One Another Passionately and Alleviate Suffering". We must also attempt to live as Intelligently, Courageously, and Joyfully as possible.

- "SEMPER FI"
- "BLUE SKIES"
- "VAYA SIN DIOS"

Oh, and one more thing, No matter what you do -

DO NOT WALK INTO A TAIL ROTOR!

IMPORTANT AND USEFUL ACRONYMS

-AACN: American Association of Critical Care Nurses

-ABG: Arterial Blood Gas

-ABSNC: Accreditation Board of Specialty Nursing Certifications

-ACLS: Advanced Cardiac Life Support

-ADN: Associate Degree in Nursing

-ALOC: Altered Level of Consciousness

-AMS: Altered Mental Status

-ARDS: Acute Respiratory Distress Syndrome

-ASTNA: Air and Surface Transport Nurses Association

-BCCTPC: Board for Critical Care Transport Paramedic Certification

-BCEN: Board of Certification for Emergency Nurses

-BGL: Blood Glucose Level

-BLS: Basic Life Support

-BSI: Body Substance Isolation

-BSN: Bachelors of Science in Nursing

-BVM: Bag Valve Mask

-CAMTS: Commission on Accreditation of Medical Transport Systems

-CBS: Clinical Base Supervisor

-CBS: Community Based Service

-CCP: Cerebral Perfusion Pressure (Brain)

-CCP: Coronary Perfusion Pressure (Heart)

-CCRN: Critical Care Registered Nurse

-CCT: Critical Care Transport

-CCU: Cardiac Care Unit

-CEN: Certified Emergency Nurse

-CFIT: Controlled Flight Into Terrain

-CFRN: Certified Flight Registered Nurse

-CHF: Congestive Heart Failure

-CMS: Circulation, Motor, Sensation

-C-NPT: Certification in Neonatal Pediatric Transport

-CO: Cardiac Output

-COPD: Chronic Obstructive Pulmonary Disease

-CPEN: Certified Pediatric Emergency Nurse

-CPR: Cardiopulmonary Resuscitation

-CRM: Crew Resource Management

-CRFS: Crash Resistant Fuel Systems

-CSF: Cerebrospinal Fluid

-CTRN: Certified Transport Registered Nurse

-CVP: Central Venous Pressure (Preload)

-CXR: Chest X-ray

-DAI: Drug Assisted Intubation (RSI)

-DIC: Disseminated Intravascular Coagulation

-DKA: Diabetic Ketoacidosis

-DOU: Direct Observation Unit

-DL: Direct Laryngoscope

-ELT: Emergency Locator Transmitter

-ENA: Emergency Nurses Association

-ENPC: Emergency Nursing Pediatric Course

-ETCO2: End Tidal CO2

-ETT: Endotracheal Tube

-FBO: Fixed Base Operator (Aviation Fueling Station)

-FDGB: Fall Down Go Boom

-FIO2: Fraction of Inspired Oxygen

-FW: Fixed Wing (Jet and Propeller Airplanes)

-GSW: Gun Shot Wound

-HBS: Hospital Based Service

-HEMS: Helicopter Emergency Medical Services

-HR: Heart Rate

-IABP: Intra-Aortic Balloon Pump

-IBSC: The International Board of Specialty Certification

-IC: Incident Commander / Incident Command

-ICP: Intracranial Pressure

-IFR: Instrument Flight Rules (Double-Engine Birds (If outfitted))

-IFT: Interfacility Transport

-IIMC: Inadvertent Instrument Meteorological Condition

-IO: Intraosseous

-IV: Intravenous

-JIC: Just In Case

-LBRT: Length Based Resuscitation Tape

-LLE: Left Lower Extremity

-LT: Left

-LUE: Left Upper Extremity

-LVN: Licensed Vocational Nurse

-LZ: Landing Zone

-MAP: Mean Arterial Pressure

-MCA: Motorcycle Accident

-MCI: Mass Casualty Incident

-MEL: Minimum Equipment List

-MI: Myocardial Infarction

-MICU: Medical Intensive Care Unit

-MSA: Minimum Safe Altitude

-MVC: Motor Vehicle Collision

-NCC: National Certification Corporation

-NCLEX-RN: National Council Licensure Examination for Registered Nurses

-NCSBN: National Council of State Boards of Nursing

-NGT: Nasogastric Tube

-NICU: Neonatal Intensive Care Unit

-NoTAM: Notice to Airmen

-NPO: Nothing Per Oral

-NRP: Neonatal Resuscitation Provider

-NVG: Night Vision Goggles

-OCD: Obsessive Compulsive Disorder

-OGT: Orogastric Tube

-PALS: Pediatric Advanced Life Support

-PAP: Pulmonary Artery Pressure

-PAWP: Pulmonary Artery Wedge Pressure

-PEEP: Positive End-Expiratory Pressure

-PIC: Pilot In Command

-PICU: Pediatric Intensive Care Unit

-PM: Paramedic

-PNA: Pneumonia

-PNCB: Pediatric Nursing Certification Board

-PRN: As Needed

-Pt: Patient

-PTX: Pneumothorax

-R&D: Research and Development

-REBOA: Resuscitative Endovascular Balloon Occlusion of the Aorta

-RLE: Right Lower Extremity

-RSI: Rapid Sequence Intubation (DAI)

-RR: Respiratory Rate

-RT: Respiratory Therapist

-RT: Right

-RUE: Right Upper Extremity

-RW: Rotor Wing (Helicopter)

-SBP: Systolic Blood Pressure

-SCIWORA: Spinal Cord Inj w/o Radiographic Abnormality

-SICU: Surgical Intensive Care Unit

-SIVP: Slow IV Push

-SMR: Spinal Motion Restriction (Spinal Precautions)

-STEMI: S-T Elevation MI

-STN: Society of Trauma Nurses

-SVR: Systemic Vascular Resistance (Afterload)

-TBI: Traumatic Brain Injury

-TCAS: Traffic Collision Avoidance System

-TFBR: Throttle, Fuel, Battery, Rotor (Post Crash Shutoff Sequence)

-TFR: Temporary Flight Restriction

-TNCC: Trauma Nursing Core Course

-TPATC: Transport Provider Advanced Trauma Course

-TV (or VT): Tidal Volume

-TXA: Tranexamic Acid

-UNICEF: United Nations Children's Fund

-VE: Minute Ventilation

-VFR: Visual Flight Rules (Single-Engine Birds)

-VL: Video Laryngoscope

-WCS: Worst Case Scenario

-WHO: World Health Organization

RECOMMENDED BOOKS

ASTNA; Renee S. Holleran; Allen C. Wolfe; Michael A. Frakes

Patient Transport: Principles and Practice

Renee S. Holleran

Mosby's CEN Exam Review

&

Mosby's Emergency & Transport Nursing Exam Review

Orchid Lee Lopez

Back To Basics: Critical Care Transport Certification Review

William E. Wingfield

The Aeromedical Certification Examinations Self-Assessment
Test

Samuel M. Galvagno

Emergency Pathophysiology - Clinical Applications for
Prehospital Care

Hildy M. Schell; Kathleen A. Puntillo

Critical Care Nursing Secrets

Laura Gasparis Vonfrolio; Joanne Noone

Critical Care Examination Review

(CCRN study book- aka- The "Vonfrolio Green" Book)

&

Emergency Nursing Examination Review

(CEN study book -aka- The "Vonfrolio Purple" Book)

ENA

Certified Pediatric Emergency Nurse (CPEN) Review Manual

Eric R. Bauer

FlightBridgeED, LLC - FP-C/CFRN Certification Review &
Advanced Practice Update

&

F.A.S.T Exam Prep: FlightBridgeED - Air - Surface - Transport -
Exam - Prep & Ventilator Management: A Pre-Hospital
Perspective

Scott DeBoer

Certified Pediatric Emergency Nurse Review: Putting It All
Together

&

Peds Pearls: Tear-Out Tips, Tricks & Treasures from the
Trenches

Charles F. Swearingen

Swearingen's Resource and Study Guide for Critical Care Transport Clinicians

&

Vent Hero: Advanced Transport Ventilator Management

BCEN; Ann J. Brorsen

TCRN Certification Review

Kendra Menzies Kent

Trauma Certified Registered Nurse (TCRN) Examination Review: Think in Questions, Learn by Rationales

----

Kyle Faudree

Flight Paramedic Certification - A Comprehensive Study Guide

William Owens

The Ventilator Book

&

The Advanced Ventilator Book

James Michael Rich

SLAM: Street Level Airway Management

Ron M. Walls; Michael F. Murphy; Calvin A. Brown III; John C. Sakles; Nathan W. Mick

The Walls Manual of Emergency Airway Management

John B. West

Respiratory Physiology - The Essentials

UMBC

Critical Care Transport Field Guide

Informed; Jon Tardiff; Paula Derr

Emergency & Critical Care Pocket Guide

Paul Maxwell

Mosby Jems' Rapid Rescue Spanish

Janice Hudson

Trauma Junkie: Memoirs of an Emergency Flight Nurse

David M. Kaniecki

Operation Flight Nurse: Real-Life Medical Emergencies

Kevin Hazzard

A Thousand Naked Strangers: A Paramedic's Wild Ride to the Edge and Back

----

Sonja Schwartzbach

Oh Sh*t! I Almost Killed You! - A Little Book of Big Things Nursing School Forgot to Teach You

----

James R. Stein Jr.

Doin It With The Lights On - Exploits of a Paramedic

Mary Hart

Tough Lessons - A Flight Nurse Learned How to Manage Turbulence In The Air and In Her Life, and You Can Too!

Samuel Shem

The House of God

Pat Jensen

Shock Trauma

Richard Dawkins

The Greatest Show on Earth

Christopher Hitchens

Mortality

Sam Harris

Waking Up

Neil de Grasse Tyson

Astrophysics for People in a Hurry

Ayaan Hirsi Ali

Infidel

Stephen Hawking

The Universe in a Nutshell

Bill Bryson

A Short History of Nearly Everything

Sun Tzu

The Art of War

ABOUT THE AUTHOR

Nurse Rob still works full-time in Flight/Transport Nursing. He lives in San Diego, California and enjoys Skydiving, Scuba Diving, Shred Guitar Playing, Brazilian Jiu Jitsu, Science Promotion, Sailing, Traveling, and Relaxing with his Kittens and his muse, Miss Jennie.

Please feel welcome to contact him with any questions or invite him to lecture or motivationally speak at your workplace, conference, or event.

Made in the USA
San Bernardino, CA
15 August 2020